Strength Training for Men

A special thank you to Strength and Conditioning Coaches Peter Valabek and Michal Hrcka for assisting with the development of this book.

The Body Coach Series

# Strength Training for Men

## The Ultimate Core Strength to Power Conversion Training System

Paul Collins

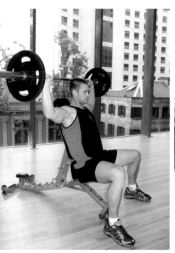 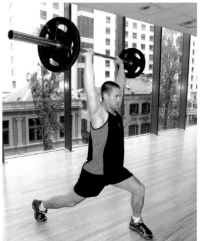 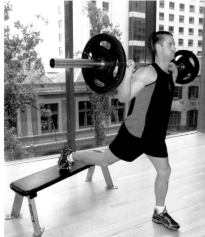

Meyer & Meyer Sport

British Library Cataloguing in Publication Data
A catalogue record for this book is available from the British Library

Paul Collins
**Strength Training for Men**
Maidenhead: Meyer & Meyer Sport (UK) Ltd., 2010
ISBN 978-1-84126-286-4

© 2010 Paul Collins (text & photos)
and Meyer & Meyer Sport (UK) Ltd. (Layout)
Aachen, Adelaide, Auckland, Budapest, Cape Town, Graz, Indianapolis,
Maidenhead, Olten (CH), Singapore, Toronto
 Member of the World
Sport Publishers' Association (WSPA)
www.w-s-p-a.org

Printed and bound by: B.O.S.S Druck und Medien GmbH, Germany
ISBN 978-1-84126-286-4
E-Mail: info@m-m-sports.com
www.m-m-sports.com

# Contents

## Trademarks

Body Coach®, The Body Coach®, Fastfeet®, Quickfeet®, Speedhoop®, Posturefit®, Spinal Unloading Block®, Australia's Personal Trainer™, Speed for Sport™, Collins-Technique™, Coach Collins™, Collins Lateral Fly™, 20-40-60 Exercise Principle™, 3B's Principle™ , Personal Training for Pets™, PT for Pets™ are trademarks of Paul Collins.

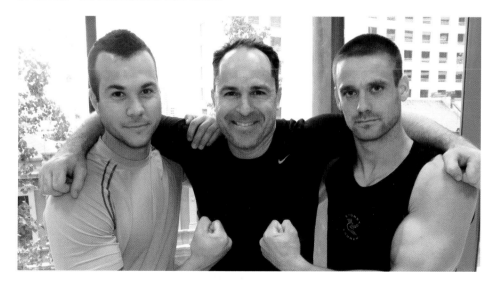

Body Coach® Team – Peter, Paul und Michal

## About the Author

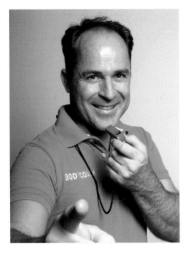

Paul Collins, Australia's Personal Trainer™ is founder of The Body Coach® fitness products, books, DVD's and educational coaching systems – helping people to get fit, lose weight, look good and feel great. Coaching since age 14, Paul has personally trained world-class athletes and teams in a variety of sports from Track and Field, Squash, Rugby, Golf, Soccer and Tennis to members of the Australian World Championship Karate Team, Manly 1st Grade Rugby Union Team and members of the world-renowned Australian Olympic and Paralympic Swimming teams. Paul is an outstanding athlete in his own right, having played grade rugby league in the national competition, being an A-grade squash player, National Budokan Karate Champion and NSW State Masters Athletics Track & Field Champion.

A recipient of the prestigious 'Fitness Instructor of the Year Award' in Australia, Paul is regarded by his peers as the 'Trainers' Trainer' having educated thousands of fitness instructors and personal trainers and appearing on TV, radio and print media features. Over the past decade, Paul has presented to national sporting bodies including the Australian Track and Field Coaching Association, Australia Swimming Coaches and Teachers Association, Australian Rugby League, Australian Karate Federation and the Australian Fitness Industry as well as travelling to present a highly entertaining series of corporate health & well-being seminars for companies focused on a Body for Success™ in life and in business.

Paul holds a Bachelor of Physical Education degree from the Australian College of Physical Education. He is also a Certified Trainer and Assessor, Strength and Conditioning Coach with the Australian Sports Commission and Olympic Weight Lifting Club Power Coach with the Australian Weightlifting Federation. As a Certified Personal Trainer with Fitness Australia, Paul combines over two decades of experience as a talented athlete, coach and mentor for people of all age groups and ability levels in achieving their optimal potential.

In his free time, Paul enjoys competing in track and field, massage, travelling, nice food and movies. He resides in Sydney, Australia.

**For more details visit: www.thebodycoach.com**

## A Word from The Body Coach®

For any man looking at increasing his muscular strength, achieving his athletic ambitions or building his best body shape ever – *Strength Training for Men* is the perfect practical training guide for you!

*Strength Training for Men* adds a new dimension to muscular development with its revolutionary 5-Phase **Core Strength to Power Conversion Training System™** that takes the guesswork out of training and offers a unique learning experience for achieving the ultimate athletic body.

*Strength Training for Men* is loaded with exercise information for any athlete, coach or trainer at any level. It contains all the fundamental guidelines for participating in a safe and efficient strength training program, whilst sequencing exercises towards the development of more explosive power with my breakthrough 5-Phase Core Strength to Power Conversion Training System™.

I say this with confidence, as I have broken down advanced Olympic lifting techniques into individual movement patterns. With this I have devised a 5-phase training system that allows you build essential core strength and stability whilst establishing functional movement awareness of your body and at the same time progressing towards more advanced lifting. I have found that teaching Olympic lifts such as the Snatch and Clean and Jerk is much easier if you first break down each of the movements and teach them as partial stages of the entire lift whilst gaining the appropriate strength, body awareness and flexibility. Once you have mastered each individual movement and gained the appropriate foundation strength and technique, you will find performing the whole movement is much easier as you will have gradually developed the essential neuromuscular framework for optimal power performance to occur.

Just like a professional golfer learning how to perfect their golf swing, you too can increase your own training knowledge, awareness and understanding for maximizing strength and power gains in a safe, efficient and productive manner with the **5-Phase Core Strength to Power Conversion Training System™** incorporating:

1. **Strength Foundation**
2. **Core Strength Development**
3. **Complex Strength to Power Conversion**
4. **Olympic Lifting - Power Conversion**
5. **Program Design**

The major benefit of this approach lies in the progression of isolated to more complex compound movement patterns, ultimately improving Central Nervous System (CNS) recruitment, muscular coordination, fat loss and boosting testosterone levels – enhancing one's libido, muscular gains and physical and mental energy levels.

As foundation strength exercises and core strength development is progressed into more complex exercises, the body really starts to engage in strength to power conversion which provides the foundational support for more highly explosive Olympic lifting drills. With the vast array of exercises available, athletes of every level will be able to quickly learn, execute and master the movements. As a result, you will be able to improve efficiency and explosiveness each time you step into the weight room.

As a practical strength training guide, combining these 5 phases with some basic sports science and anatomy of movement I encourage you to apply the training principles outlined and progressively work between chapters to master the movements to ready yourself for athletic competition and realize your true physical performance potential. Then in the final phase I provide you with a variety of sample training programs including the Body Coach® Strength Training System and 12-Week Sports Strength and Olympic Lifting Programs as well as a 20-Week Training Plan and Nutritional Timing for Optimal Strength, Muscle Growth and Power Gains.

On top of improving your knowledge and understanding of strength training, my goal is to help you develop intramuscular coordination to increase motor-unit recruitment, firing rates and synchronization. In saying this, general hypertrophy training is important to increase the force-generation capacities of all muscles, as well as strengthening core muscles. This progresses into developing one's neural activation capacity of the relevant muscular framework in performing Olympic lifts which I've broken down for you. For those of you focused on sports improvements, just remember that the maximization of transfer to sports performance requires the conversion of powerful muscles to a specific co-coordinated sports skill, hence the importance of including powerful Plyometric type drills like you can find in my book *Power Training*. As well as time devoted to daily stretching, massage and sound nutritional and recovery practices for achieving optimal results.

I look forward to working with you!

**Paul Collins**
The Body Coach®

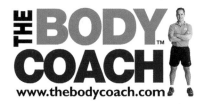

www.thebodycoach.com

# Chapter 1
## Conversion Training System

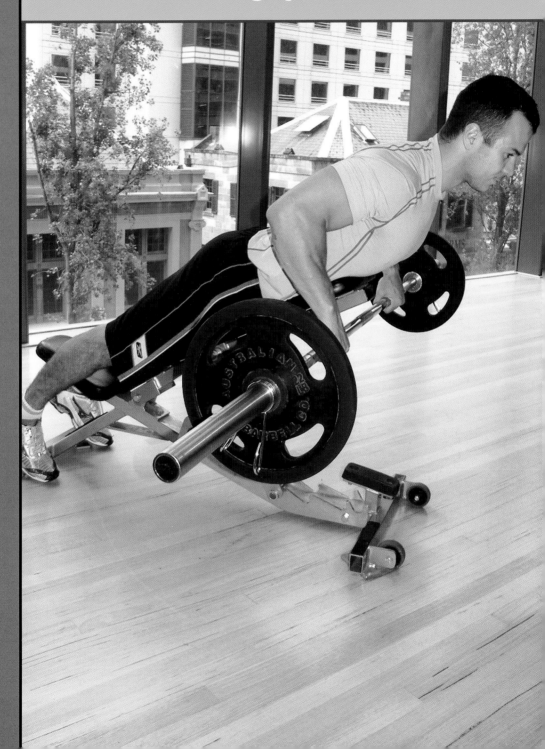

Every good exercise program starts with a method upon which training principles are based. In my book, **Awesome Abs**, I devised a 5-Phase Abdominal Training System for maximizing your core potential. In **Speed for Sport™** I devised a 6-Stage Fastfeet® Training Model for maximizing your speed potential. In **Functional Fitness** I devised a Functional Fitness Method (FFM) with '6 Key Movement Patterns' that aim to provide a balance of muscular strength, fitness and mobility throughout multiple planes of motion. Now, in **Strength Training for Men**, I have devised the **5-Phase Core Strength to Power Conversion Training System™** which aims to improve fundamental core strength, mobility and coordination required for Olympic lifting and power gains.

# 5-Phase Core Strength to Power Conversion Training System™

All athletes involved in contact or physical sports such as AFL, NBA, NFL, NHL, NRL or similar, must possess a enormous level of strength, stability and explosive power to be successful. The Core Strength to Power Conversion Training System™ provides a functional strength progression program based on the breakdown of Olympic lifting exercises – the ultimate in power development. By breaking down complex lifts into individual movement patterns, over time, as strength, coordination and mobility improve through a periodized training cycle, a functional exercise progression is applied that links two or more strength exercises together to form a functional movement pattern. This progressive training approach is aimed at allowing the muscles and joints, Central Nervous System (CNS) and other bodily systems to progressively adapt to the training stress put forth. As timing improves with functional lifting between muscle groups, strengths and weakness are balanced out, which ensures the muscles and CNS fire more rapidly allowing a higher output of power to be achieved. This innovative approach aims to help athletes avoid overtraining and burnout by working within their capabilities. It does this by taking them back a few notches in training to build the essential foundational strength from which more explosive power can be achieved in the future.

The problem we face today is that many people want to imitate their sporting heroes and how they train without any base training platform, which ultimately leads to incorrect lifting, overtraining and injury. This is what makes the Core Strength to Power Conversion Training System™ so important – by firstly showing you what you can achieve through Olympic lifting, then breaking these movements down into training phases (1-4) which provide the building blocks from which successful progression can occur. As the body adapts and becomes stronger, exercises are linked together to become complex compound strength to power conversion movements that combine multiple muscle groups. The more strength and power the higher the activation of the Central Nervous System (CNS) and the more recovery is required. These benefits themselves come with recovery in between training sessions (nutrition, supplements, rest, massage, etc.), so the linking of exercises gradually allows the body to adapt to the training stimulus from which more output can be achieved.

To bring this understanding together, imagine the electrical voltage required to light up your house compared to that of a sports stadium. Yes, they both serve the same purpose of lighting up an environment, but one requires more power voltage output than the other and stronger network and energy source in order to maintain a constant high power output and avoid failure. As most people are not elite athletes, with years and often decades of training experience, they need to understand that they need a plan to train and re-wire their bodies to enable them to build and maintain the essential strength, technique and neuromuscular feedback that will enable them to work at a higher level, without failing. If they do, their voltage and power output levels will increase appropriately if applying the 5-Phase Core Strength to Power Conversion Training System™.

# 5-Phase Training System

The innovative approach of the 5-Phase Core Strength to Power Conversion Training System™ allows athletes to breakdown complex movement patterns into individual sequences whilst at the same time allowing the body, its muscles, joints, energy and nervous systems time to progressively adapt for optimal balance and athletic performance improvement. Below are the 5 phases involved:

## Phase 1: Strength Foundation

Strength foundation training is the general preparation phase based on a diverse range of strength movement exercises that aim to improve muscle coordination and endurance and neural adaptation, before progressing onto the goal of increasing the cross-sectional area of muscle and ultimately maximum strength. The main exercises provided in Phase 1 have been adapted from the breakdown of Olympic lifting phases into individual isolated and compound exercises that target larger muscle groups used in sports and for gaining overall athleticism. It is essential that a general body weight strength base is acquired prior to and maintained throughout foundation strength training for postural support. This phase includes exercise instruction in technique and breathing for maximizing muscular fitness.

## Phase 2: Core Strength Development

Core strength of the abdominal and lower back region is important because it controls the position of the pelvis and provides the synergy between the upper and lower extremities in powerful movement. Abdominal wall musculature without adequate endurance, strength and coordination is more likely to permit surrounding tissues to be taken past their physiological limit. The muscles of the pelvic, hip and lower back region should be free of muscular tension to ensure good pelvic mobility and abdominal contraction.

## Phase 3: Complex Strength to Power Conversion

Quite simply, after developing strength (Phases 1 and 2), your goal is convert strength to power. In this phase, we concentrate on exercises that link two or more strength foundation exercises together that form a part or sequence of an Olympic lift – requiring the athlete to generate high levels of speed and force. This stage is essential in building technique and muscular coordination of more powerful lifts together with the continual adaptation of the neuromuscular framework as part of the strength to power conversion using sub-maximal loads for mastering technique before increasing the loads.

## Phase 4: Olympic Lifting – Power Conversion

The technical aspects of Olympic lifting can be practiced throughout any development stage at a lower sub-maximal intensity under the guidance of a certified strength and conditioning coach. Although, once progressing through the developmental phases of Strength Training for Men and reaching Phase 4, the appropriate building blocks in neuromuscular strength and power will have been established for full Olympic lifts (including Power Versions) to be undertaken at first sub-maximally and later near maximal levels under the guidance and supervision of a certified strength and conditioning coach. The objective is to never sacrifice your lifting technique for a heavier weight and ensure the strength foundation is in place by participating in Phases 1-4 of the Training System.

## Phase 5: Program Design

One of the most important elements of any sport or activity is a well-designed strength training program. By establishing an understanding of each training phase (1-4) and the exercises to be performed, a series of progressive strength training programs can be established to help guide you towards your goal. Appropriate gains in strength itself require the attention of a number of training variables. Being able to identify and apply the anatomy of movement on the following pages helps you progress in your complete knowledge and understanding of training requirements and optimal performance. The nutrient timing for optimal strength, muscle growth and power gains is also supplied to ensure you maximize your training outcomes and achieve the ultimate athletic body shape.

**Note:** This 5 Phase process is not designed for an Olympic lifter, instead athletes, body builders and gym enthusiasts looking at improving their training edge through a system of progressive strength to power training techniques. For this reason, if your goal is to become an Olympic lifter I encourage you to contact your national weight lifting association.

5-Phase Core Strength to Power Conversion Training System™

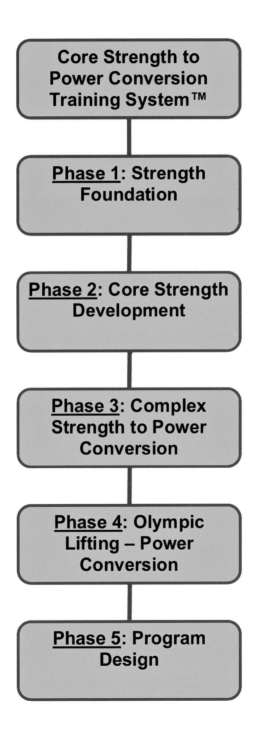

## Anatomy of Movement

Strength training has a variety of terms used to describe the movement patterns, muscle contractions and various descriptions when exercising. Simple terms often become more complex as training progresses, which can seem confusing at times, although the more you get involved the more knowledge and understanding you'll have of your body. In this chapter I will outline many of the important key words used throughout this book.

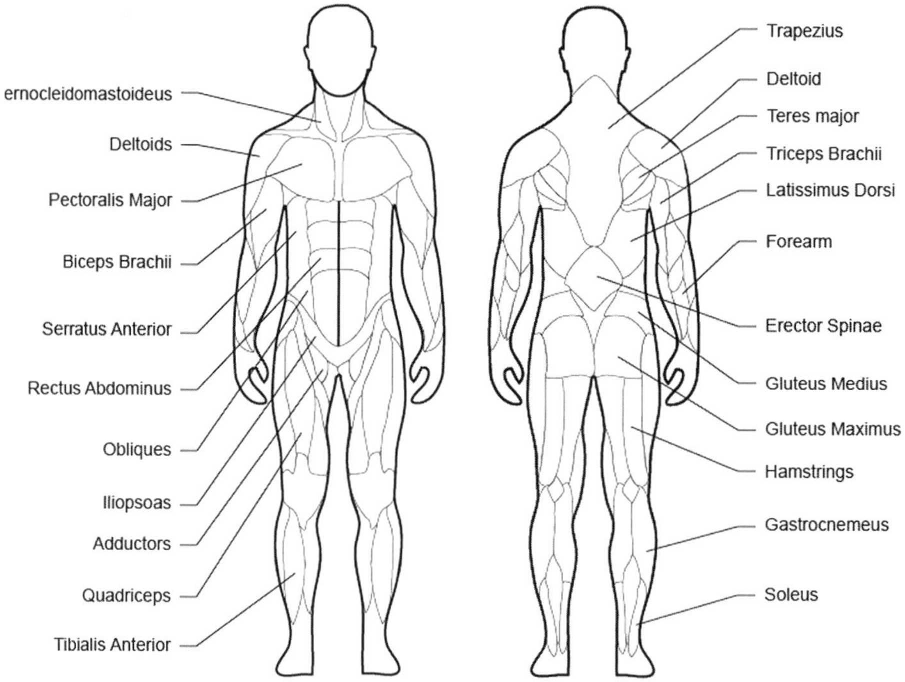
ernocleidomastoideus
Deltoids
Pectoralis Major
Biceps Brachii
Serratus Anterior
Rectus Abdominus
Obliques
Iliopsoas
Adductors
Quadriceps
Tibialis Anterior
Trapezius
Deltoid
Teres major
Triceps Brachii
Latissimus Dorsi
Forearm
Erector Spinae
Gluteus Medius
Gluteus Maximus
Hamstrings
Gastrocnemeus
Soleus

## Joint Actions

Muscular joints of the body provide a fulcrum point for muscles to be worked. There are six types of joint actions. In the table below I will describe the movement and example exercise:

| JOINT ACTION | MOVEMENT DESCRIPTION | EXAMPLE MOVEMENT |
|---|---|---|
| Flexion | Decreasing joint angle | Biceps Curl |
| Extension | Increasing joint angle | Leg Extension |
| Abduction | Movement away from the body midline | Deltoid Lateral Raises |
| Adduction | Movement toward the body midline | Horizontal Chest Flyes |
| Rotation | Rotation about an axis | Twisting the Arm |
| Circumduction | 360 degree rotation | Circling the arm around |

## Anatomical Planes

The body itself is divided into three anatomical planes – Sagittal, Frontal and Horizontal. The Sagittal plane divides the body down the center or vertically. The Frontal plane divides the body from front to back. The Horizontal plane divides upper and lower. The table below lists the anatomical terms and the corresponding descriptions.

| ANATOMICAL TERM | DESCRIPTION |
| --- | --- |
| Anterior | Front |
| Medial | Inside |
| Posterior | Rear |
| Lateral | Outside |
| Supine | Face up |
| Unilateral | One side |
| Bilateral | Both sides |
| Prone | Face down |
| Superior | Upper |
| Inferior | Lower |

**Each of the movements of the muscles of the body is described by the following terms:**
- Abductor – Moves a limb away from the midline
- Adductor – Moves a limb toward the midline
- Extensor – Increases the angle at a joint (extends a limb)
- Flexor – Decreases the angle at a joint (flexes a limb)
- Pronator – Turns a limb to face downwards
- Supinator – Turns a limb to face upwards
- Rotator – Rotates a limb

## Types of Muscle Contraction

While it is known that muscle fibers can only contract and shorten, as a whole they can develop a force in more than one way as shown below:

| | |
| --- | --- |
| **Isometric** | Where the muscle tension and muscle length remain constant |
| **Concentric** | Where the muscles shorten as the fibers contract |
| **Eccentric** | Where the muscles lengthens as it develops tension |
| **Isokinetic** | Where the muscle contracts through its full range of movement |

In each exercise there are four main functions of the associated muscles:

1. **Agonists** (prime movers) - generally refers to the muscle we are exercising.
2. **Antagonists** - is the opposing muscle and acts in contrast to the agonist.
3. **Stabilizers** - are those that hold a joint in place so that the exercise may be performed. The stabilizer muscles are not necessarily moving during exercise, but provide stationary support.
4. **Assistors** - help the Agonist muscle doing the work.

The following table lists muscles and their opposing counterparts. These columns are reversed when exercising muscle on the right hand column, for example, the Antagonist becomes the Agonist and visa versa:

| AGONIST (Prime Mover) | ANTAGONIST |
|---|---|
| Biceps | Triceps |
| Deltoids | Latissimus Dorsi |
| Pectoralis Major | Trapezius/Rhomboids |
| Rectus Abdominis | Erector Spinae |
| Iliopsoas | Gluteus Maximus |
| Hip Adductor | Gluteus Medius |
| Quadriceps | Hamstrings |
| Tibialis Anterior | Gastrocnemius |

In prescribing all 5 phases in Strength Training for Men, it is important to have muscle balance to prevent injury. Muscular balance refers to the relationship between the Agonist and Antagonist. If the Agonist is much stronger than the Antagonist (or visa versa) the Agonist can overpower the Antagonist and cause injury.

## Exercise Terminology
Exercise terminology is generated separated into 3 key areas:
1. **Isolated** – is an exercise that involves just one discernible joint movement.
2. **Compound** – relates to an exercise that involves two or more joint movements.
3. **Static** – refers to holding a muscle in a static position relative to the desired body position.

# 3B's Principle™: Pre-exercise Set-up

Every exercise has a number of key elements to consider when setting up and performing a movement. Applying correct technique from the onset will help establish good form which is ultimately maintained until the repetitions or set is completed. After reviewing Anatomy of Movement, the key elements required in order to maintain good body position whilst exercising form part of a simple exercise set-up phrase I've termed the **3B's Principle™**:

## 1. Brace
Activating and bracing your abdominal muscles whilst exercising is important because it helps increase awareness of your body position as well as helping unload any stress placed on the lower back region.

## 2. Breath
In foundation and core strength training, you breathe out when you exert a force – such as pushing the bar up and extending the arms in the bench press exercise or rising up straight from a squat position. You then breathe in with recovery – such as lower the bar towards the chest with the bench press exercise or lowering the body and bending the legs when performing a squat. Breathing should remain constant throughout each exercise.

## 3. Body Position
To complete the 3B's Principle™, the third B relates to one's ability to hold a good body position and technique with each exercise. In all exercises, ensure good head and neck, spine and pelvic alignment is maintained at all times with the rest of the body. The overall focus of each exercise should therefore be on quality of the movement.

So, next time you perform any exercise, simply apply the 3B's Principle™ from start to finish in order to maintain correct technique and body posture to help maximize strength gains.

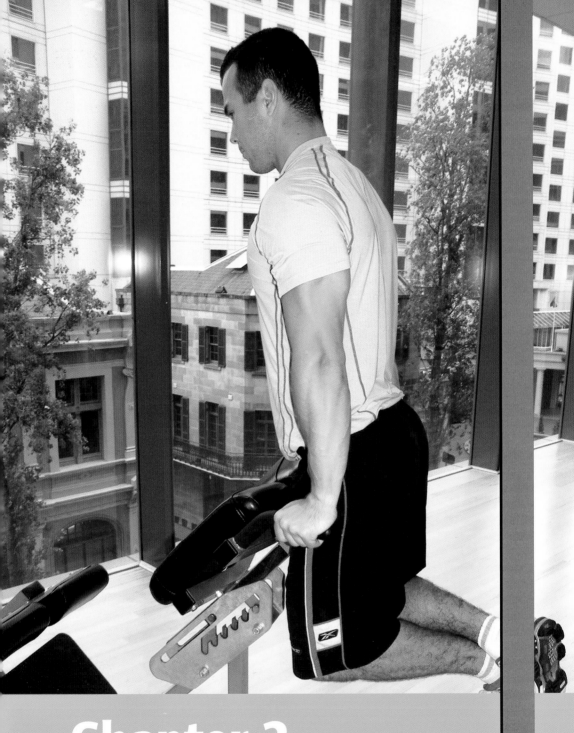

# Chapter 2

**Phase 1: Strength Foundation**

Strength training is a key component for success in many sports and physical activities. In Phase 1, the objective is to develop a solid foundation of strength by focusing on enhancing one's muscular framework through a progressive overload towards exerting a maximal force against a resistance using mainly free weights and various machines.

This chapter focuses on key exercises for improving muscular gains for the chest, triceps, shoulders, back, biceps and forearms, upper and lower back, gluteus, hamstrings, quadriceps and calves. Exercises include both isolated single joint and compound multi-joint exercises. Many of the exercises within this chapter also form part of Phase 3 development exercises and can be referred back to for reference purposes.

If you are new to strength training, returning after a long break or willing to take time to learn how to train effectively – then foundation strength training is a great starting point for you as it initiates the progressive resistance and overload principle. On the other hand, if you have a strong training background over many years you may simply use Phase 1 as a reference guide to refer too especially when working through Phase 3. Either way both will benefit and should work through this chapter to grasp all training phases within this book.

## Progressive Resistance Training

In any physical activity, your muscles grow in response to the challenge placed upon them. Over time the muscles adapt to this stimulus and require an additional challenge for muscular strength gains to occur. The stimulus for this to occur evolves around **eight key elements**, some of which work simultaneously together, including:

| 8 Key Elements | Description |
|---|---|
| 1. Exercise Intensity | Weight (or mass) being lifted; based upon a percentage of one's maximum lift or 1RM (repetition maximum) used by advanced athletes and coaches for establishing training loads, reps and sets |
| 2. Speed of Movement – Repetition Ratio | Speed ratio of concentric and eccentric movement as well as mass being lifted – i.e. slow, fast or a combination of both, for example 3:1:1 Ratio (or 3 seconds eccentric, 1 second transition, 1 second concentric) used in hypertrophy. Variations of these ratios apply, which can manipulate the intensity. |
| 3. Time Muscle Is Under Tension | Number of repetitions being performed; speed of movement and the exercise intensity |
| 4. Type of Exercise | Actual exercise and movement being performed for specific muscle group – as there are many variations for each muscle group |
| 5. Volume of Work | Total number of repetitions and sets being performed as well as the frequency |
| 6. Rest Periods | Recovery period between exercises and sets can dictate fatigue or regeneration |
| 7. Frequency | How often you train |
| 8. Mental Focus | How much effort and focus you put into your training session |

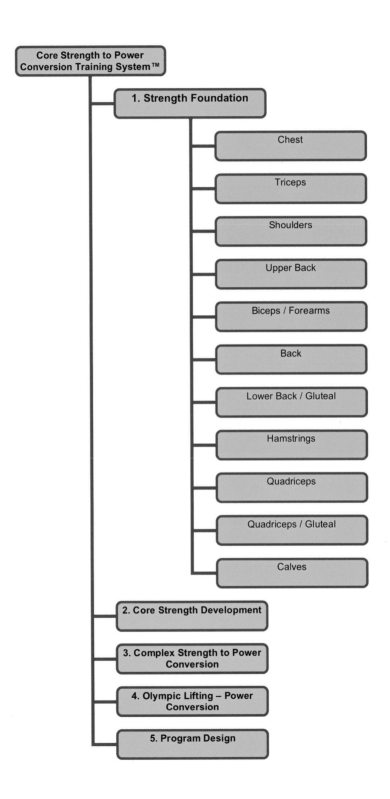

In strength training, variations of these eight key elements play a major role in the outcome of your training. Many people can lift weights for years without change to their body shape or strength levels. So, to help take you to a new level in your training knowledge, understanding and approach, we utilize the Foundation Strength Training Zone Chart. This training guideline is aimed at helping you understand the training zone you need to work on in order to improve your strength and your goals. Along the journey, there is a little work to be done by regularly adapting and applying the eight key elements as part of the Foundation Strength Training Zones.

| Foundation Strength Training Zones | Repetition Range | Percentage of 1RM | Training Effect |
|---|---|---|---|
| 1. Muscle Endurance<br><br>**Phases 1–2**<br>Please note: All percentages act as a guide only, as these may vary slightly with more specific and detailed training programs | 12-20+ reps | 40-60% | Aimed at developing a muscle's ability to contract over an extended period. Primarily for use are Phases 1-2 of Strength Training for Men to allow the muscles, tendons and joints of the body time to adapt as part of a general preparation phase all athletes must acquire |
| 2. Muscle Hypertrophy<br><br>**Phases 1–2** | 8-12 reps | 60-80% | Aimed at solely increasing the cross-sectional area of the targeted muscle. In many instances, better results come from a slower speed of movement ratio for each repetition. Primarily for use are Phases 1-2 of Strength Training for Men. |
| 3. Maximal Strength<br><br>**Phases 1–3** | (i) 6-8 reps<br>(ii) 4-6 reps | 80-85%<br>85-90% | Aimed at increasing one's neuromuscular efficiency, strength and coordination between muscle groups. In many instances, better results come from a faster speed of movement without technique breakdown. Primarily for use are Phases 1-3 of Strength Training for Men. |

| 4. Power Conversion | (i) 1-5 reps | 87.5-100% | Aimed at transferring maximal strength gains by increasing the speed at which you apply a force using more complex exercises such as Olympic Lifting. Primarily for use are Phases 3-4 of Strength Training for Men. |
| | (ii) 1-3 reps | 92.5-100% | |

**Phases 3–4**
Note: In some instances a lighter weight (and percentage) is used and rapid movement pattern applied for more sports specific power conversion.

**Outcome:** Each strength training zone targets the two specific skeletal muscle tissue fibers in different ways. Consisting of both slow twitch (aerobic oriented) and **fast twitch** (anaerobic) contracting muscle fibers, the speed and intensity at which you train manipulates how the muscles respond and work together. As muscle fibers blend together the **slow twitch** element responds generally to low power production and resistance to fatigue, whereas fast twitch fibers which have low fatigue resistance respond to high power production important in power sports and sprinting. This helps dictate the training cycles you undertake in order to build a strength foundation (Phase 1-2) and more powerful foundation (Phases 3-4) using a Periodization Plan.

In most instances, no one training model fits all. So, think of this chart like a tree without branches. What I'm providing you with here is a training model that provides a benchmark for you to apply, but as you grow so do your branches (just like that of a tree) and variables of the strength training zones need to be adjusted, adapted and manipulated from the eight key elements. For instance, a simple adjustment of the speed of movement can make dramatic changes to the training intensity. A common mistake often made by athletes is moving the bar or performing an exercise too fast. Here's an example:

If your goal is to build your chest region and you were performing 8 reps in 8 seconds (1 second a rep) on the bench press, the time the muscle is under tension is minimal compared to if I asked you to perform each repetition using a 3:1:1 ratio – 3 seconds lowering, 1-second transition/hold and 1 second explosion upwards with bar (for a 5-second repetition x 8 reps = 45-seconds under tension). Whilst strength gains may occur performing faster repetitions, increasing the cross-sectional area or size of a muscle works best following the 3:1:1 ratio – or its variations such as 3:0:1 or 2:0:1 and so forth. In saying this, a faster speed may be used at certain times within a training plan to suit your training goals. This is where our training process called periodization fits into the equation.

## Periodization Plan

To help maximize one's performance all year round, we transfer the foundation training zone chart phases into a scheduled training cycle called periodization. This process allows an athlete to plan yearly, quarterly, monthly, weekly and even daily the type of training they will perform in order to work towards peaking for an event or series of events. Within this framework, training loads and volumes (sets, reps, percentage of maximum lifts) are manipulated in order to achieve specific training goals. The scientific nature of this training approach relates to the specific requirements of each sport. For a seasonal athlete, a training cycle may consist of a 12-month period involving an off-season (transition) phase, pre-season and competition phases. This annual training plan is subdivided into periods of time to suit these phases for improving strength, fitness or speed over a period of time. This is referred to as macro-cycles, for example, a preparatory phase may consist of 16 weeks; within this 16-week period it may be broken down into 4 x 4-week cycles (macro-cycles) that build up in intensity towards the competition phase. Within a macro-cycle are smaller weekly cycles called micro-cycles that are used to plan daily training sessions. The benefit of a periodization plan is that it provides a training plan platform for improvements in strength, maximum strength and power to occur. In a sporting environment where multiple physical components such as speed, fitness, strength and agility and skills sessions are required in parallel the periodization plan allows you plan each session as well as recovery. Think of it like attending school or college where you have a yearly class schedule broken down into terms or semesters with holiday breaks in between. Along the way there is regular testing just like playing competitive sport before a final exam (or final series). Below is a general example of how a periodization plan may look. These will vary for each sport:

| Training Phases | Pre-season | | Competition | | Transition | |
|---|---|---|---|---|---|---|
| Macro-cycles | 4-weeks | | | | | |
| Micro cycles | | | | | | |

## Linear and Non-Linear Training Approach

In *Strength Training for Men*, we start off with a linear training approach of 'Core Strength to Power Conversion' which involves establishing a strength foundation (training base), improving technique and muscle fiber response whilst working towards maximal power output from performing Olympic lifts. The linear training approach involves decreasing the volume and increasing the intensity each week in order to maximize strength, power or combination of both. There are many variables that can be used. Here is one example:

- Weeks 1-4:          1 x 12-15 reps
- Weeks 5-8:          2 x 10-12 reps
- Weeks 9-12:         3 x 8-10 reps
- Weeks 13-16:        4 x 6-8 reps

A **non-linear approach** alternating between phases of higher volume and higher intensity throughout a cycle can also be applied for more advanced athletes and those within a competitive period. For instance, a non-linear approach maybe performed over 3-4-week cycles or within a weekly cycle itself, for example: Monday low intensity (12-15 reps); Wednesday high intensity (6-8 reps) and Friday moderate intensity (10-12) reps. Below are three periodization cycle samples combining the above approaches into 8-16-week training cycles:
(1) 16-week periodization model for the beginner
(2) 12-week periodization model for the intermediate and more advanced
(3) 8-week advanced training cycle

**Note:** With multiple training variables existing, the following samples provide a baseline training approach for you to build a greater knowledge, awareness and understanding of training cycles and how your body responds. You may find some elite athletes or coaches may criticize or be negative towards such cycles, but just remember everyone has a starting point from which they will have once progressed and built upon – just like these. So, once you have hands-on experience in the gym and successfully worked through these training cycles (Phases 1-5, the 8-Key Elements and Periodization plan), you too can make specific adaptations and modifications to your training program with an approach that best suits your training needs and what you found works best for you.

## 16-Week Beginner's Cycle
This cycle is designed for the beginner, 'gym–goer' or athlete returning to training after a lengthy lay-off – as the first 4-weeks are important in preparing the muscles, tendons and joints for the training cycles ahead and reducing the risk of injury. This general model is broken down into 4-week progressive cycles. After 4 weeks of initial training, the percentage of 1RM is established under the guidance of a professional strength and conditioning coach and used as a guideline throughout each 4-week cycle, namely weeks 5-16, where it is re-tested.

| | |
|---|---|
| Weeks 1-4 | Muscle endurance utilizing exercises from Phases 1–2 |
| Weeks 5-8 | Muscle hypertrophy utilizing exercises from Phases 1–2 |
| Weeks 9-12 | Maximum strength utilizing exercises from Phases 1 & 3 |
| Weeks 12-16 | Power conversion utilizing exercises from Phases 1, 3, 4 |

## 12-Week Intermediate to Advanced Cycle
In this cycle, an intermediate to advanced level athlete or trainer will have already established a sound training base for the support structures and starts with hypertrophy approach in weeks 1-4 before progressing.

| | |
|---|---|
| Weeks 1-4 | Muscle hypertrophy utilizing exercises from Phases 1–2 |
| Weeks 5-8 | Maximum strength utilizing exercises from Phases 1 & 3 |
| Weeks 9-12 | Power conversion utilizing exercises from Phases 1, 3, 4 |

## 8-Week Advanced Training Cycle
In this cycle, an advanced athlete can apply rotating cycles of high and medium intensity exercise over 3-weeks followed by a light CNS week that before transition into a new 4 week training cycle. The objective is focused on in-season training cycles for the advanced athlete that can be modified to suit their training goals and competition schedule accordingly.

| | |
|---|---|
| Weeks 1-4 | Maximum strength utilizing exercises from Phases 1 & 3 |
| Weeks 5-8 | Power conversion utilizing exercises from Phases 1, 3, 4 |

Throughout the 8, 12 and 16 week cycles, core strength (Phase 2) is maintained varying the loads, reps, sets and speed of movement to ensure a strong mid-section is maintained all year round. For more specific abdominal core exercises refer to my Body Coach® books on Abdominal Training, Power Training and Core Strength.

The initiative throughout each 4-week training cycle is to gradually increase the volume (sets, reps and frequency) and intensity (described here as a percentage of your 1-Repetition Maximum – 1RM) to allow you to work towards a peak level. In some instances you may extend the cycle by an extra week or two also applying a low, medium and high intensity schedule. As every sport is unique it is important to work alongside a professional strength and conditioning coach to design the best periodization plan for you!

Rest and recovery also plays a significant role during each training cycle with many athletes performing a light week of training during the final week of each phase as a transition into the next one. Rest is also important for growth and development of the muscles throughout each training week to allow muscle fibers and energy systems to adapt and recover to avoid overtraining and injury. For more specific training programs refer to Phase 5 page XX. It is also recommended to work with a professional strength and conditioning coach in the proper development of a periodization plan designed specifically for your needs.

## Repetition Maximum (RM) Testing

Intensity in exercise is most easily represented as a percentage of one's maximum lift. Establishing this maximal percentage is important in the overall training model as it provides a benchmark from which your training loads and repetitions are based. One of the most universally accepted methods for testing strength and power is the 1RM or the maximum amount of weight the athlete can lift for no more than one complete repetition of that strength related exercise. This method allows you to determine the loads used throughout the training program and is generally only applied to compound (multi-joint) exercises such as:

* Bench Press (page 30)
* Squat (page 62-63)
* Dead-Lift (page 56)
* Power Clean (page 107)

A minimum 4-8 week training base is required prior to attempting any repetition maximum tests to ensure that the muscle, joints and tendons have adapted and proper technique has been established. This test should only be performed under the guidance of a professional strength and conditioning coach for accuracy and safety reasons. Most importantly, this can be re-tested throughout the training cycle as a tool that allows one to gauge whether to increase or decrease one's training load.

Now before I go any further I'd like you to recognize that performing a 1RM attempt is not the preferred method for a beginner, but an elite athlete or Olympic lifter, because of the high intensity and risk level. Instead, working with a weight that can be lifted for 5 repetitions (5RM) which equates to approximately 87.5% of your maximum from which a 1RM can be calculated, is the preferred method.

## Testing Method

To begin, start with a cardiovascular warm-up and light stretch. This is followed by a warm-up set of 12 repetitions of the specific exercise to be tested using a light weight. Rest for 60-seconds whilst increasing the weight to perform 8 repetitions followed by 120-second rest.

With your strength and conditioning coach, estimate what you believe your 5 repetition maximum weight will be. This means that you can only just complete a 5th rep and not 6 reps. If attempting the 5RM and you only complete 3 reps or so, rest for 180 seconds before attempting with a lighter weight.

**Bench Press 5RM Example:** (after initial cardiovascular warm-up)

1. Bench press warm-up exercise performing 12 reps of light weight.
2. Rest 60-seconds.
3. Bench press warm-up exercise performing 8 reps of medium weight.
4. Rest 120-seconds.
5. Bench press with estimated 5RM weight.
6. If too easy or too heavy and more or less repetitions completed, rest for 180 seconds before repeating this test with new estimated weight.
7. Once correct, multiply the 5RM (as 87.5% of your 1RM) as shown in calculation below:

**Example of 5RM lift of 95kg (210 lbs.) into a 1RM:**

$$\frac{100}{87.5} \times \text{weight lifted} = \frac{100}{87.5} \times 95kg = 108kg \text{ (rounded off to 105kg)}$$

Once a 1RM can be established, training loads for various repetitions in training can also be established. Note: The smallest weight increments in heavy lifts are generally 2.5kg on both sides of the bar, equating to 5kg combined. If whilst performing a 5RM, only 4.5 reps are completed you could generally announce that a reduction of 5kg off the total weight you could perform for 5 reps. Always round off your total score to a zero (0) or 5 number (ie. 100kg or 105kg or 110kg and so forth). Note: 1 kilogram (kg) = 2.2 pounds (lbs.)

**Estimating Training Loads**

| 1rep | 2reps | 3reps | 4reps | 6reps | 8reps | 10reps | 12reps |
|------|-------|-------|-------|-------|-------|--------|--------|
| 100% | 95% | 92.5% | 90% | 85% | 80% | 75% | 65% |

For an advanced or elite athlete the 1RM specific test maybe performed using a similar example as above with lighter weights and higher reps followed by recovery period before increasing weight and reducing the reps near maximal loads.

Quite often when you transfer a 1RM score into a workout schedule (i.e. 3 sets of 12 reps at 65% of 1RM) you may find that you are able to perform 1 or 2 sets easy and unable to complete the third. This is when you know you are on the right track, because as your strength and muscle endurance improves and you are able to complete 3 sets easily, then the weight being lifted must be increased. On the other hand, if 65% is initially too hard this may need to be reduced to what your body tells you (ie. 55-60%). Remember, these tables only act as a guideline from which you can adapt your training model.

**Note:** Refer to Phase 5 for sample strength training programs (page 157)

## Isolated and Compound Movements

All exercises vary in their movement mechanics. **Isolated** exercises refer to single joint exercises that target a specific muscle group, for example, the biceps arm curl exercise (elbow joint) specifically targets the biceps muscle group of the upper arm. On the other hand, **compound** exercises involve more than one joint such as movement at the ankle, knee, and hip with an exercise such as a squat. In most instances, the larger muscle groups incorporating larger muscle groups should always form the basis of your routine. Common compound movements are squats, presses, pull-ups, push-ups, and rows, as well as the Olympic lifts and their assistance exercises (such as pulls, presses, shrugs on toes, etc.).

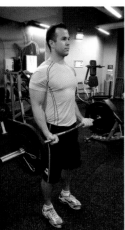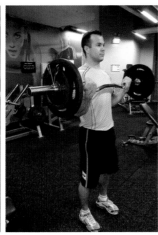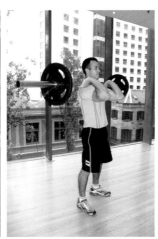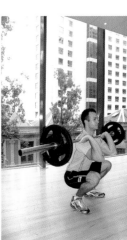

**Isolated Exercise – Biceps Curl**                    **Compound Exercise – Squat**

Ideally more difficult movements which use many joints and muscles are placed first in the workout, while simpler isolated exercises which move only one joint (such as biceps curls or leg extension) are placed towards the end. Usually exercises for torso musculature (abdominals, obliques, lower back) are also placed at the end in order to ensure that they are fresh for more demanding exercises in the beginning, and able to provide as much torso support as possible. Otherwise the abdominal muscles can have their own separate training routine as shown in Phase 2.

## Strength Training Guidelines – A Few Rules!

Now by this point you can see how complex training can become and why athletes have coaches so they can specifically focus on training and competing alone. Below are a few rules to be applied for any exercise being performed:

- Always gain approval to exercise by your doctor and physical therapist.

- It is important during this phase that a proper warm-up, cool down and stretching routine is adapted to ensure effective range of motion is maintained and improved. Spend 5-10 minutes increasing heart rate through aerobic activity such as:

## Warm-up Drill Examples include:

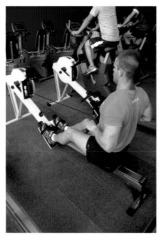
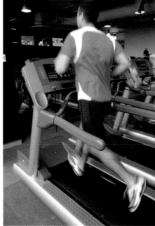
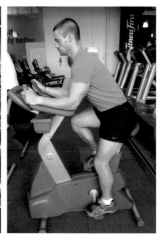

Rowing                    Jogging                    Cycling

- Stretching is recommended before, during and after exercise with a major focus on stretches being held for longer periods after training.
- Each exercise should be preceded by a warm-up set using a light resistance (50-60%) for the specific exercise that follows.
- Apply 3B's Principle™ – Brace, Breath and Body Position with each exercise.
- Utilize the hook grip (as shown below) on all pulling exercises.
- Always maintain good posture and body alignment by focusing on the exercise at hand.
- Maintain deep breathing throughout each exercise. Breath in on recovery and breath out when exerting a force.
- Never sacrifice your lifting technique for a heavier weight.
- Always train under the guidance of certified strength and conditioning coach, Olympic lifting coach or personal trainer.
- Always cool down and stretch after lifting.
- Apply the principles of Nutrient Timing for Optimal Strength Gains on page 173.
- Always apply the 8-Key Elements (p.19) when training as part of your training progression.
- Ensure you drink plenty of water – before during and after training.

## Applying the Hook Grip

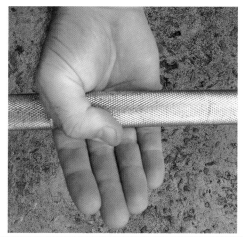
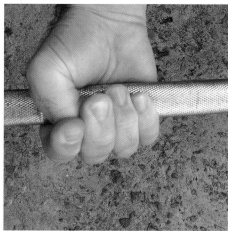

| 1. Thumb across Bar | 2. Apply Hook Grip |

The hook grip is the key grip used in all pulling exercises such as the Dead-Lift, Snatch and other similar movements – some in part or full movement. The hook grip is employed to ensure the firmest possible non-slip grip on the barbell and should be initiated from the beginning in all training. Initially it will feel uncomfortable but overtime will become an integral part of your lifting mechanics.

Below you will find exercises used to strengthen each muscular region of the body:

## Chest

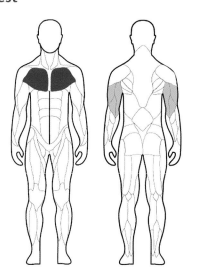

**MUSCLES WORKED**

■ **PRIMARY**
Chest

■ **SECONDARY**
Triceps

- Pectoralis (Chest) – Large fan shaped muscle that covers the front of the upper chest.
- Triceps – The rear side of the upper arm.

## Bench Press

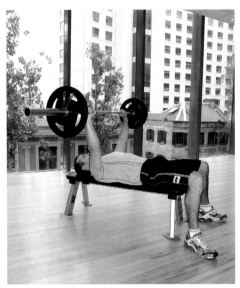

Start

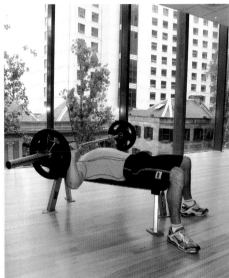

Midpoint

### Instruction

- Lie on your back on flat bench.
- Grip bar evenly slightly wider than shoulder-width apart.
- Maintaining the natural curve of your lower back, brace your stomach.
- Breathe in as you lower the barbell towards the midline of your chest.
- Breathe out as you press the barbell to arm's length.
- Maintain a continuous flowing movement at all times until repetitions are completed.

**Note:** The closer the grip, the more triceps involvement.

In all exercises that follow, ensure you continually refer back to the 8-Key Elements (page 19) as part of your training guide in order to maximize your training goals.

## Incline Bench Press

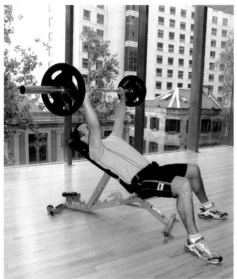 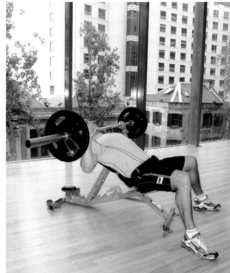

Start                                                    Midpoint

### Instruction

- Lie on your back on incline bench.
- Grip bar evenly slightly wider than shoulder-width apart.
- Maintaining the natural curve of your lower back, brace your stomach.
- Breathe in as you lower the barbell to the midline of your chest.
- Breathe out as you press the barbell to arm's length.
- Maintain a continuous flowing movement at all times until repetitions are completed.

## Incline Dumbbell Chest Press

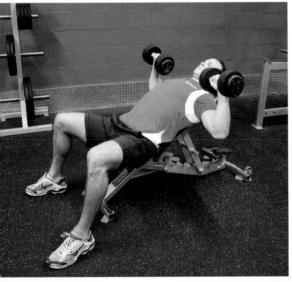 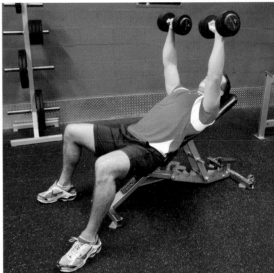

| Start | Midpoint |

### Instruction

- Lie on your back on incline bench.
- Rest dumbbells in hands evenly above shoulder level with arms at 90-degrees.
- Breathe out as you press the dumbbells overhead to arm's length and bring together.
- Breathe in as you lower the dumbbells to starting point.
- Maintain a continuous flowing movement at all times until repetitions completed.

**Note:** This exercise can be performed on a flat or incline bench.

# Dumbbell Chest Flyes

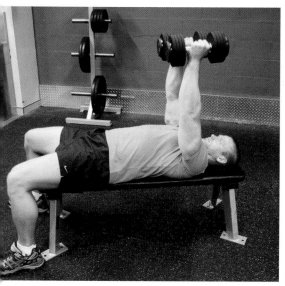 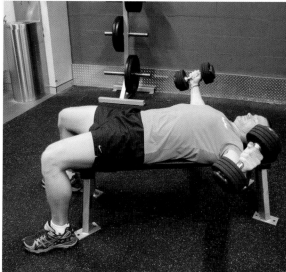

| Start | Midpoint |
|-------|----------|

## Instruction

- Lie on your back on flat bench.
- With dumbbells in hand, extend arms above head with palms facing together and arms slightly bent.
- Breathe in as you slowly lower the dumbbells out to side, maintaining the arms in a slightly bent position at all times.
- Breathe out as you raise the dumbbells back up to arm's length and bring together.
- Maintain a continuous flowing movement at all times until repetitions are completed.

**Note:** This exercise can be performed on a flat or incline bench.

# Triceps

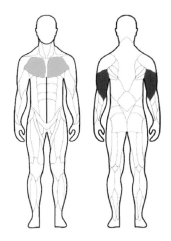

**MUSCLES WORKED**

■ **PRIMARY**
Triceps

■ **SECONDARY**
Chest

- Triceps – The rear side of the upper arm.
- Pectoralis (Chest) – Large fan-shaped muscle that covers the front of the upper chest.

## Lying Triceps Extension

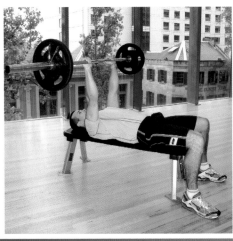
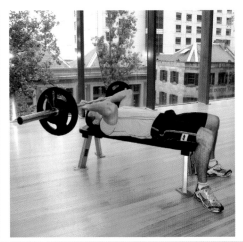

Start                                           Midpoint

### Instruction

- Lying on flat bench, grip barbell shoulder-width apart with an overhand grip (palms facing towards you).
- Extend arms above chest level.
- Keeping the natural curve of your lower back, brace your stomach.
- Breathe in as you slowly lower the bar toward your forehead, bending your elbows and leading with your knuckles.
- Breathe out as you return the barbell to arm's length.
- Keep the barbell moving at all times in an even and controlled manner in time with your deep breathing.

# Arm Dips

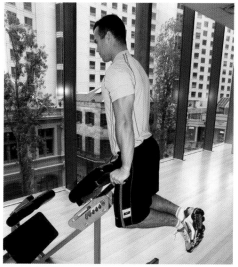 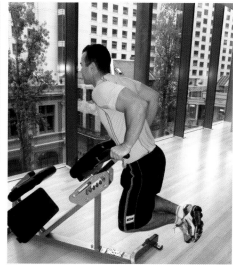

Start                                                    Midpoint

## Instruction

- Rise up onto parallel bars and extend arms.
- Ensure shoulders and head are kept high to avoid sinking and good body position is maintained.
- Breathe in and lower the body, leaning the chest slightly forward until the arms reach a 90 degree angle (no lower).
- Breathe out and raise body – keeping the arms close to body as they extend.
- Keep the movement flowing at all times in an even and controlled manner in time with your deep breathing.

**Note:** This exercise also incorporates chest involvement as will many other triceps exercises.

## Triceps Push Down

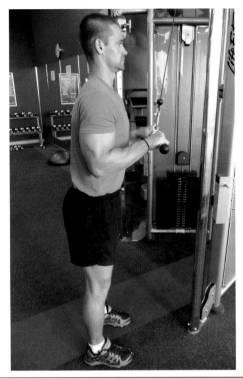 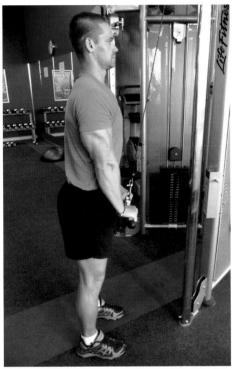

Start         Midpoint

### Instruction

- Stand one step back from cable machine and grip flat (or V-shaped) handle.
- Keep arms close to the side with elbows bent at 90 degrees.
- Maintaining the natural curve of your lower back, brace your stomach.
- Breathe out as you push the handle down to straighten the arms.
- Breathe in as you control the handle, keeping the arms close to the body back to 90-degree angle.
- Maintain a continuous flowing movement at all times until repetitions are completed.

## Standing Overhead Triceps Extension

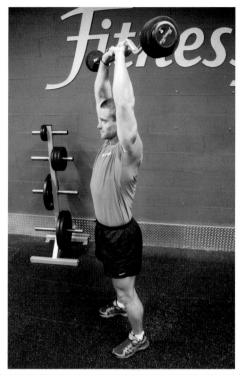 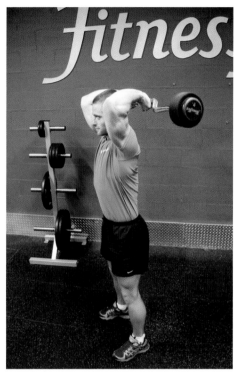

| Start | Midpoint |
|---|---|

### Instruction

- Stand tall gripping ezy-bar (or straight bar) overhead with hands close together.
- Maintaining the natural curve of your lower back, brace your stomach.
- Breathe in as you lower the barbell by bending the arms and lowering behind the head.
- Breathe out as you press the barbell back to arm's length overhead.
- Maintain a continuous flowing movement at all times until repetitions are completed.

**Note:** This exercise can also be performed in a standing lunge position (one leg forward and the other back) with the abdominals braced to avoid any lower back arching with the weight overhead.

# Shoulders

The deltoid (shoulder) muscle covers the shoulder and consists of three distinct segments:

1. The anterior or front deltoid allows you to raise your arm to the front.
2. The medial or middle deltoid allows you to raise your arm to the side.
3. The posterior or rear deltoid allows you to draw your arm backwards when it is perpendicular to the torso.

Different exercise movements of the shoulder region target the different heads of the deltoid.

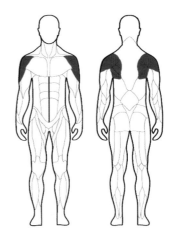

**MUSCLES WORKED**

■ **PRIMARY**
Shoulders

■ **SECONDARY**

## Seated Front Shoulder Press

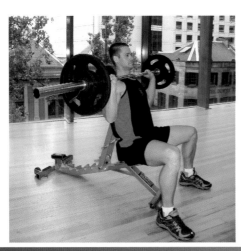 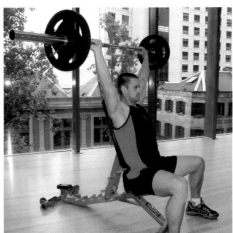

| Start | Midpoint |
|-------|----------|

## Instruction

- Sit on upright bench with your back straight, head in line with your spine and feet shoulder-width apart.
- Grip barbell across front of shoulders, hands shoulder-width apart.
- Maintaining the natural curve of your lower back, brace your stomach.
- Breathe out as you press the barbell to arm's length overhead.
- Breathe in as you lower the barbell in front of body to shoulder height.
- Maintain a continuous flowing movement at all times until repetitions are completed, resisting any arching of the lower back.

**Note:** This exercise can be performed seated or standing (Military Press) with barbell or dumbbells.

# Seated Rear Shoulder Press

- Sit on upright bench with your back straight, head in line with your spine and feet shoulder-width apart.
- Grip barbell behind head, hands wider than shoulder-width with elbows at 90-degree angle.
- Maintaining the natural curve of your lower back, brace your stomach.
- Breathe out as you press the barbell to arm's length overhead.
- Breathe in as you lower the barbell behind the head.
- Maintain a continuous flowing movement at all times until repetitions are completed, resisting any arching of the lower back.

**Note:** This exercise can be performed seated or standing.

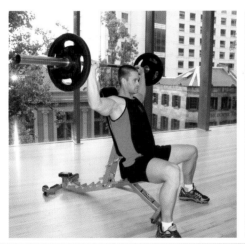 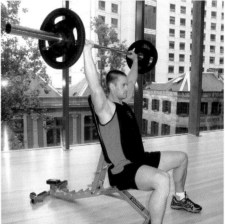

| Start | Midpoint |

## Standing Military Press

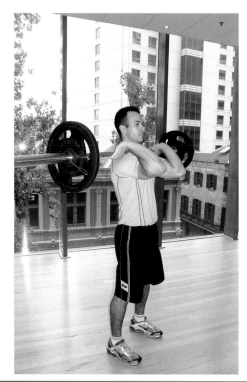
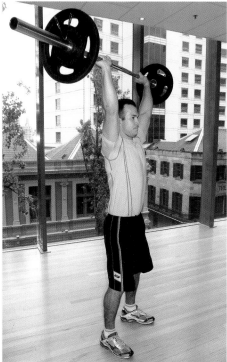

Start                                  Midpoint

## Instruction

- Stand tall resting barbell across front of shoulders with elbows high and hands shoulder-width apart.
- Maintaining the natural curve of your lower back, brace your stomach.
- Breathe out as you press the barbell to arm's length overhead.
- Breathe in as you lower the barbell in front of the body to shoulder height.
- Maintain a continuous flowing movement at all times until repetitions are completed, resisting any arching of the lower back.

**Note:** This exercise can also be performed standing in a lunge position. It also progresses into a push-press exercise using the legs to drive the bar up overhead.

# Lateral Raises

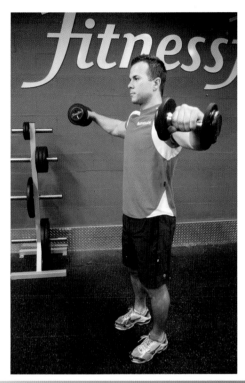

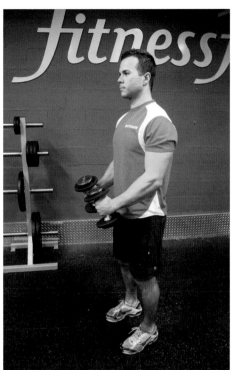

Start | Midpoint

## Instruction

- Stand tall with dumbbells in hand in front of body with arms slightly bent.
- Maintaining the natural curve of your lower back, brace your stomach.
- Breathe out as you raise the slightly bent arms up to the side until parallel to the ground – leading with the elbows.
- Breathe in as you lower the arms back down in front of the body.
- Maintain a continuous flowing movement at all times until repetitions are completed.

# Upper Back

- **Trapezius** – Upper portion of the back, sometimes referred to as 'traps' (upper trapezius) is the muscle running from the back of the neck to the shoulder.

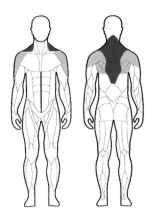

**MUSCLES WORKED**

■ PRIMARY
Upper Back

■ SECONDARY
Shoulders

## Shoulder Shrugs

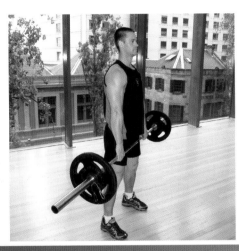

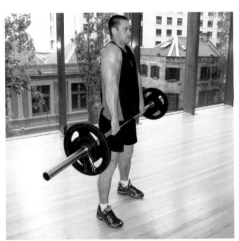

| Start | Midpoint |

### Instruction
- Stand tall gripping barbell at arm's length with hands and feet shoulder-width apart – resting bar across thighs.
- Maintaining the natural curve of your lower back, brace your stomach.
- Droop shoulders down as much as possible to start.
- Breathing out, raise shoulders up high keeping the arms straight.
- Breathe in as you lower the arms back down in front of the body.
- Maintain a continuous flowing movement at all times until repetitions are completed.

**Note:** As you raise the shoulders, you can also rotate them up and back, going in a semicircular motion from front to rear. Then slowly return to the starting position. This exercise can also be performed with dumbbells.

# Upright Row: Close, Medium, Wide & Snatch Grip

## Instruction

- Stand tall gripping barbell with overhand grip (close, medium, wide) or hook (Snatch) grip in front of body at arm's length.
- Maintaining the natural curve of your lower back, brace your stomach.
- Breathe out as you raise the bar up leading with elbows, keeping wrists straight and elbows as the highest point
- Breathe in as you lower the barbell in front of body to arm's length.
- Maintain a continuous flowing movement at all times until repetitions are completed.

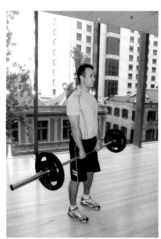
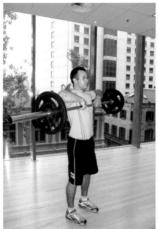

**Medium Grip** Start       **Midpoint**

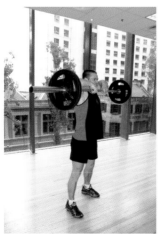
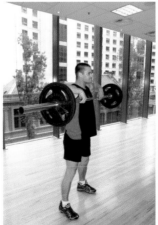
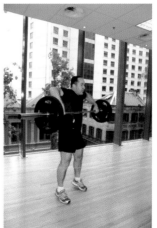

**Close Grip**       **Wide Grip**       **Snatch Grip**

## Biceps /Forearms

- **Biceps** – The front side of the upper arm which bends and supinates the elbow.
- **Forearms** – Collective muscle between the elbow and wrist bends the elbow, which pronates and supinates the elbow depending on the starting position.

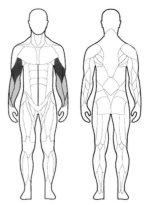

**MUSCLES WORKED**

■ **PRIMARY**
Biceps

■ **SECONDARY**
Forearms

## Barbell Biceps Curl

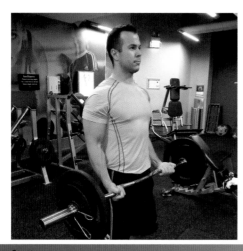
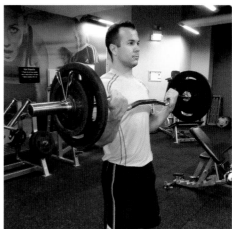

| Start | Midpoint |
|---|---|

### Instruction

- Stand with your back straight and feet shoulder-width apart, knees slightly bent.
- With your hands shoulder-width apart, take an underhand grip on barbell and rest on the front of your thighs.
- Tuck you upper arms into your body, whilst keeping your wrists straight.
- Maintaining the natural curve of your lower back, brace your stomach.
- Breathe out as you bend your elbows and draw the bar up to shoulder height – keeping your elbows close to the body.
- Breathe in as you lower the bars to your thighs.
- Maintain a continuous flowing movement at all times until repetitions completed, resisting any arching of the lower back.

**Note:** This exercise can be performed with a curl or straight bar and with feet parallel or in a lunge position.

# Alternate Arm Biceps Curl

- Stand with your back straight and feet shoulder-width apart, knees slightly bent.
- Grip dumbbells at arm's length at side of body.
- Tuck your upper arms into your body, whilst keeping your wrists straight.
- Breathe out as you bend your elbow and draw one dumbbell up to shoulder height, twisting the dumbbell as you raise your arm with palms facing towards body.
- Breathe in as you lower the dumbbell back to the side of your body.
- Repeat with opposite arm.

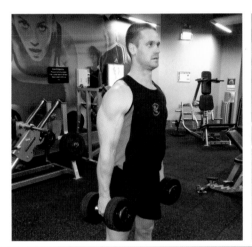 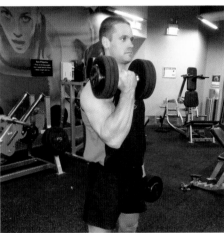

Start                                              Midpoint

**Note:** This exercise can be performed seated or standing using a single arm or both arms simultaneously.

# Back

- **Latissimus dorsi** – Large muscles of the mid-back. When properly trained they give the back a nice V shape, making the waist appear smaller. Exercise examples include pull-ups, chin and pull downs.

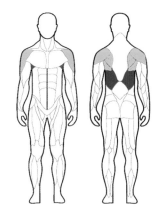

**MUSCLES WORKED**

■ **PRIMARY**
Mid-Back

■ **SECONDARY**
Shoulders

## Lat Pull Down - Front

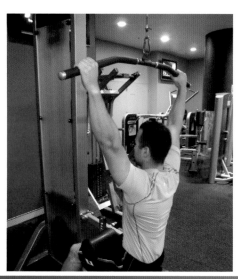
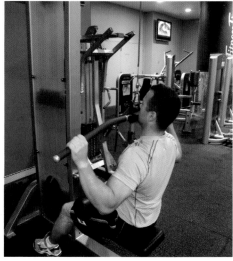

| Start | Midpoint |

### Instruction

- Take an overhand grip on wide bar overhead, wrists straight.
- Sit with your back straight, chest lifted and head in line with your spine.
- Maintaining the natural curve of your lower back, brace your stomach.
- Breathe out as you pull the bar down towards your chest by leaning slightly backwards.
- Breathe in as you allow the bar to return to upright position in a controlled manner.
- Keep the movement flowing at all times in an even and controlled manner in time with your deep breathing.

# Close Grip Pull down

- Take an overhand grip on close-grip handle overhead, wrists straight.
- Sit with your back straight, chest lifted and head in line with your spine.
- Maintaining the natural curve of your lower back, brace your stomach.
- Breathe out as you pull the handle down towards your chest by leaning slightly backwards and keeping elbows close to the body.
- Breathe in as you allow the handle to return to upright position in a controlled manner.
- Keep the movement flowing at all times in an even and controlled manner in time with your deep breathing.

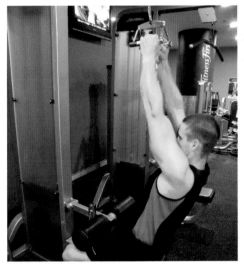 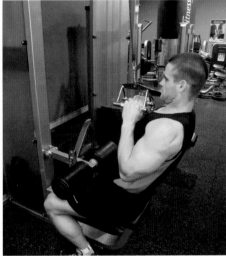

Start                                                                 Midpoint

## High Bench Pulls

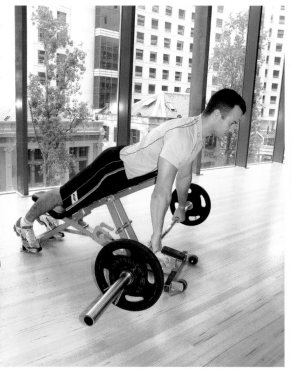 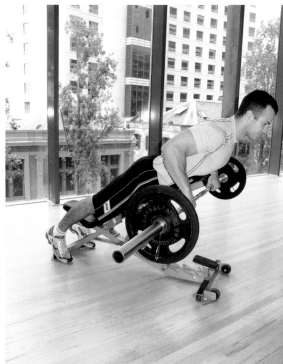

| Start | Midpoint |
|---|---|

### Instruction

- Lie face down on bench with arms extended down gripping barbell, hands shoulder-width apart.
- Maintaining the natural curve of your lower back, brace your stomach.
- Breathe out as you bend your elbows and draw the bar up towards the chest/bench – keeping your elbows close to the body.
- Breathe in as you lower the bar to full extension.
- Maintain a continuous flowing movement at all times until repetitions are completed.

**Note:** This exercise can be performed on an incline or high bench. A seated row machine exercise can be performed as a pre-requisite in strength foundation prior to the high bench pull or bent over row exercise.

# Bent Over Row

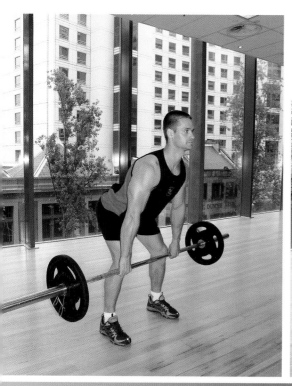 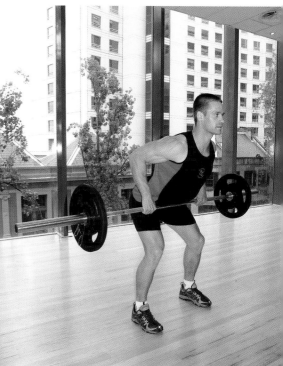

Start                                                    Midpoint

## Instruction

- Stand tall gripping barbell at arm's length with hands and feet shoulder-width apart – resting bar across thighs.
- Bend at the knees and hip region and slightly lean forwards with bar extending down over knees and directly under shoulders.
- Maintaining the natural curve of your lower back, brace your stomach.
- Tuck you upper arms into your body, whilst keeping your wrists straight.
- Breathe out as you pull bar straight up to your chest keeping elbows close to the body.
- Breathe in as you lower the bar.
- Maintain a continuous flowing movement at all times until repetitions are completed, resisting any arching of the lower back.

## Single Arm Row

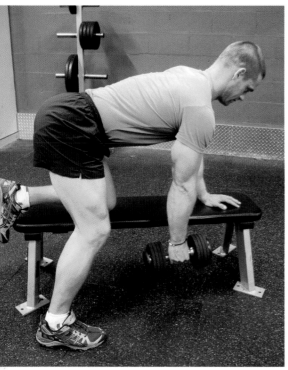 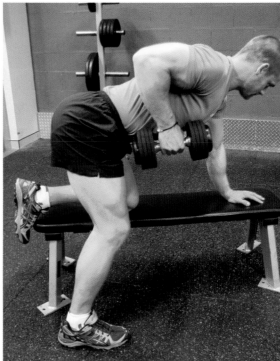

| Start | Midpoint |
|-------|----------|

### Instruction

- Place your left knee and left hand on the bench, with your hand directly in-line with your shoulder, keeping your back flat and right arm extended down gripping dumbbell.
- Maintaining the natural curve of your lower back, brace your stomach.
- Breathe out as you pull the dumbbell up toward your chest by bending your elbow – keeping your elbow close to your body at all times.
- Breathe in as you lower the dumbbell to arm's length.
- Maintain a continuous flowing movement at all times until repetitions are completed.
- Repeat movement with opposite arm with opposite leg and hand on bench.

# Chin-ups

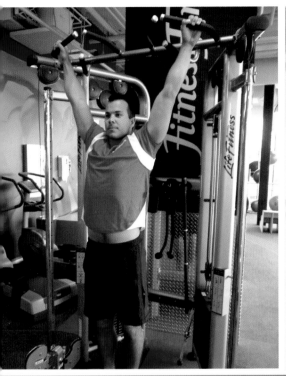

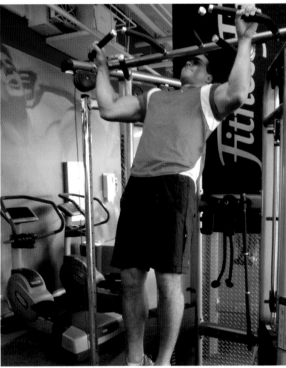

| Start | Midpoint |

## Instruction

- Take an overhand grip on bar overhead (palms facing away from you), with hands shoulder-width apart.
- Maintaining the natural curve of your lower back, brace your stomach.
- Breathe out as you pull your body upwards leading chin towards bar.
- Breathe in as you lower the body in a controlled manner to the extended starting position.
- Maintain a continuous flowing movement at all times until repetitions are completed.

## Lower Back/Glutes

- **Gluteal Region** – Often referred to as the buttock region, the primary function is hip extension in unison with the hip stabilizers important in all lower body movements.
- **Lower Back** – There are several muscles in the lower back (lumbar region) that assist with rotation, flexibility and strength. It generally refers to the segment of the torso, between the diaphragm and the sacrum on the rear side of the body from which muscle and fascia attach.
- **Hamstrings** – This is the group of muscles on the backside of the leg, running from the hip joint to the knee joint. Their primary function is to facilitate flexion of legs, medial and lateral rotation; important for walking, running and jumping.

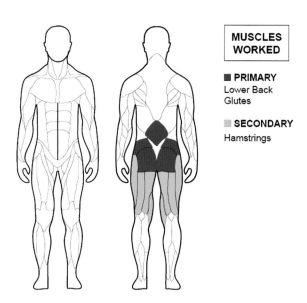

**MUSCLES WORKED**

■ **PRIMARY**
Lower Back
Glutes

■ **SECONDARY**
Hamstrings

# Romanian Dead-Lift

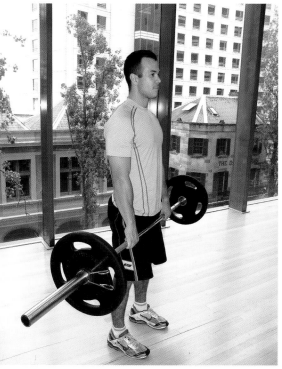

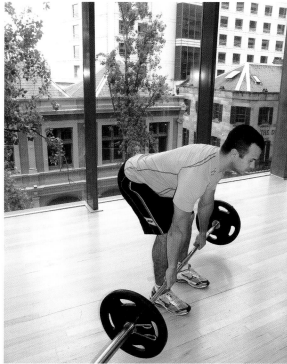

**Start**                                                    **Midpoint**

## Instruction

- Stand tall gripping barbell at arm's length with hands and feet shoulder-width apart – resting bar across thighs with legs slightly bent at the knees.
- Maintaining the natural curve of your lower back, brace your stomach.
- Breathing out, lower bar towards ground without touching, keeping arms straight and flexing at the hip.
- Breathe in as you raise back up.
- Maintain a continuous flowing movement at all times until repetitions are completed, resisting any arching of the lower back.

## Back Raises

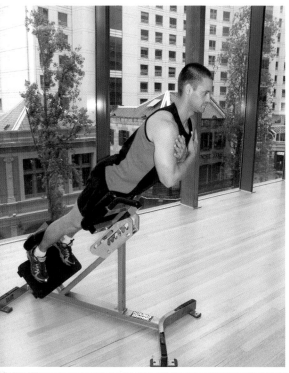

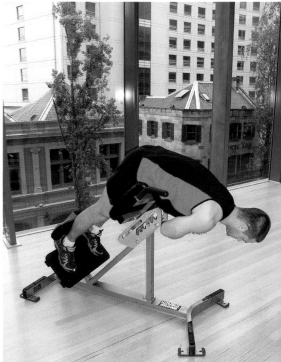

Start        Midpoint

### Instruction

- Lie face down on hyperextension bench tucking heels under foot pads.
- Adjust supporting pad height under thigh region, allowing room to bend forward at the waist without restriction.
- Cross arms across chest (with or without a weight for extra resistance).
- Maintaining the natural curve of your lower back, brace your stomach.
- Breathe in as you bend and lower forwards from the hip keeping your back flat (neutral) – avoid rounding.
- Breathe out and rise back up to starting position.
- Maintain a continuous flowing movement at all times until repetitions are completed and avoid overarching when rising.

**Note:** This exercise can also be performed resting a barbell across shoulders for more advanced athletes. Back raising machines will vary (adjust accordingly).

## Good Mornings

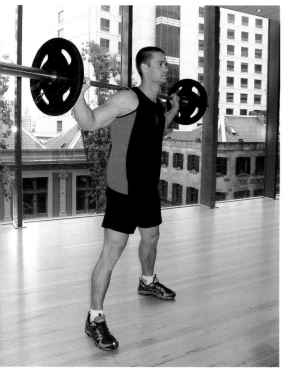 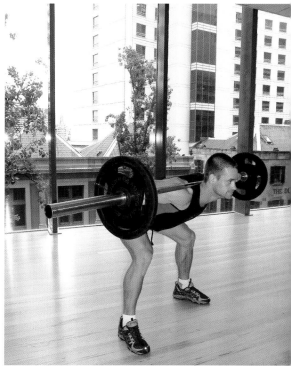

Start                                        Midpoint

### Instruction

- Stand tall with feet wider than shoulder-width apart resting barbell across rear of shoulders.
- Maintaining the natural curve of your lower back, brace your stomach.
- Breathe in as you lower forwards bending from the waist – keeping your back flat (neutral) at all times and slightly bending the knees until torso is parallel to the floor.
- Breathing out as you rise back up to starting position.
- Maintain a continuous flowing movement at all times until repetitions are completed, resisting any arching of the lower back.

**Note:** This exercise can be performed with legs slightly bent (beginner and intermediate level) or straight (more advanced level).

## Dead-Lifts

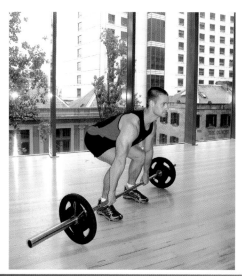 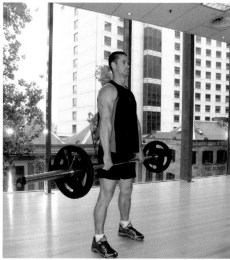

Start                                        Midpoint

### Instruction

- With barbell resting on ground, lower body into start position with feet slightly angled out approximately shoulder-width apart; shins close to the bar; knees and hip bent and arms extended holding bar slightly wider than shoulder-width outside knee alignment. Think hips, higher than knees but lower than shoulders – whilst arms are straight and extended down.
- Maintaining the natural curve of your lower back, brace your stomach.
- Breathe out as you simultaneously rise – straightening knees and hip region – into an upright standing position. During the lift, the bar will travel as close to the leg and shins as possible.
- If the hips rise before the shoulders, it means you are using your back rather than your legs. If so, reduce weight and perform exercise correctly before progressing. In this movement, most of the weight will be on the heels of the feet to help facilitate maximal contribution of the glutes and hamstrings.
- Breathe in as you rise back up to starting position reversing the lowering position simultaneously.

**Note:** Quite often as the weight gets heavier, an alternate grip is used with one palm of hand facing towards you and the other palm facing away. Alternatively wrist straps are often used with the conventional grip.

# Snatch Grip Dead-Lift

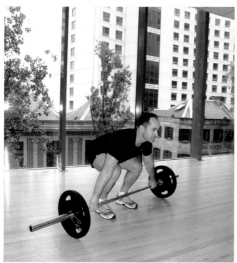 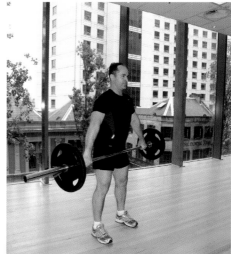

| Start | Midpoint |

## Instruction

- With barbell resting on ground, lower body into start position with feet slightly angled out approximately shoulder-width apart; shins close to the bar; knees and hip bent and arms extended out wide holding the bar utilizing a hook grip (thumb under forefingers). Think hips, higher than knees but lower than shoulders – whilst arms are straight and extended down.
- To ensure correct hand width position on bar, simply raise arms to side and bend elbows down to 90-degrees; lower down to the bar; hook grip then straighten arms.
- Maintaining the natural curve of your lower back, brace your stomach.
- Breathe out as you simultaneously rise – straightening knees and hip region – into an upright standing position. During the lift, the bar will travel as close to the leg and shins as possible.
- If the hips rise before the shoulders, it means you are using your back rather than your legs. If so, reduce weight and perform exercise correctly before progressing. In this movement, most of the weight will be on the heels of the feet to help facilitate maximal contribution of the glutes and hamstrings.
- Breathe in as you rise back up to starting position reversing the lowering position simultaneously.

# Hamstrings

- **Hamstrings** – This is the group of muscles on the backside of the leg, running from the hip joint to the knee joint. Their primary function is to facilitate flexion of legs, medial and lateral rotation; important for walking, running and jumping.

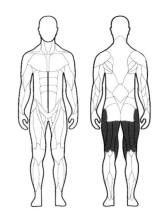

MUSCLES WORKED

■ PRIMARY
Hamstrings

▨ SECONDARY

## Leg Curl

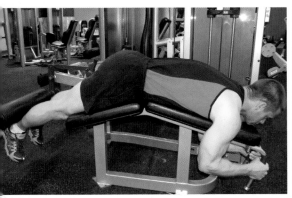

Start

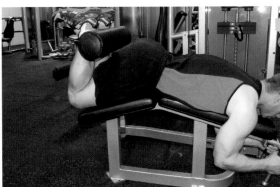

Midpoint

## Instruction

- Lie face down with lower calf and heel region placed under roller pad.
- Maintaining the natural curve of your lower back, brace your stomach.
- Breathe out as you bend your knees and curl your feet toward your buttocks – keeping your hips firmly on the bench.
- Breathe in as you lower your legs towards starting position.
- Avoid the weighted stack touching or body relaxing.
- Maintain a continuous flowing movement at all times until repetitions completed.

**Note:** This exercise can also be performed with one leg at a time.

## Glute-Ham Holds

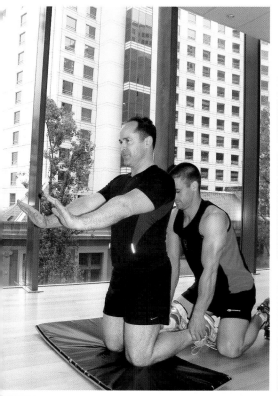

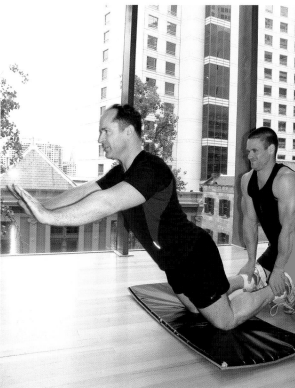

| Start | Midpoint |

### Instruction

- Kneel on ground with partner holding ankles firmly.
- Maintaining the natural curve of your lower back, brace your stomach.
- Extend arms forward of body for safety and catch into front support.
- Lean body forward and hold for set period of time eg. 2-5 seconds before lowering.
- Maintain deep breathing in and out at all times.
- Repeat drill at varying angles for set periods to strengthen hamstrings.

## Quadriceps

- **Quadriceps** – This is the large group of muscles on the front of the upper leg, often referred to as the thighs – starting at the hip joint and ending at the knee joint. Their primary function is to flex the hip and extend the knee; very important in walking, running, jumping, climbing and pedaling a bike.

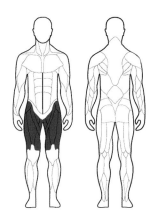

**MUSCLES WORKED**

■ PRIMARY
Quadriceps

■ SECONDARY

## Leg Extension

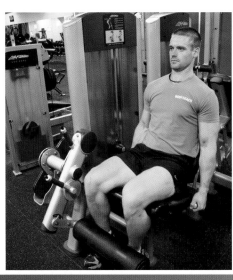 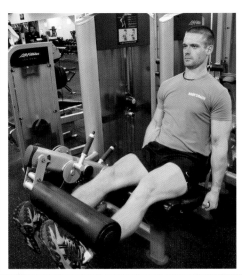

| Start | Midpoint |

### Instruction

- Sit in leg extension machine with shin region resting against pads – adjust accordingly – and flex feet by pulling toes up – whilst gripping handles (machine specific).
- Adjust back rest so bent legs (back of knee) are resting on edge of seat.
- Maintaining the natural curve of your lower back, brace your stomach.
- Breathe out as you extend the legs forward until straight.
- Breathe in as you lower your legs down – bending the knees.
- Maintain a continuous flowing movement at all times until repetitions are completed.

# Single Leg Extension

## Instruction

- Sit in leg extension machine with shin region resting against pads – adjust accordingly – and flex feet by pulling toes up – whilst gripping handles (machine specific).
- Adjust backrest so bent legs (back of knee) are resting on edge of seat.
- Maintaining the natural curve of your lower back, brace your stomach.
- Breathe out as you extend one leg forward until straight.
- Breathe in as you lower your leg down – bending the knees.
- Maintain a continuous flowing movement at all times until repetitions are completed.
- Repeat with opposite leg.

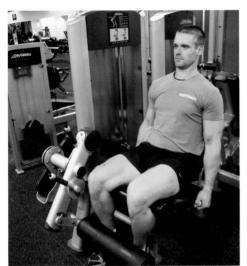 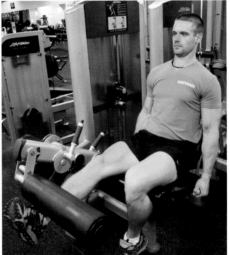

Start                                        Midpoint

## Quadriceps/Glutes/Hamstrings

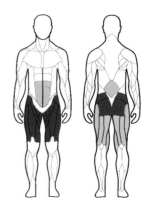

**MUSCLES WORKED**

■ **PRIMARY**
Quadriceps
Glutes

■ **SECONDARY**
Hamstrings
Abdominals
Lower Back

- **Gluteal Region** – Often referred to as the buttock region, the primary function is hip extension in unison with the hip stabilizers important in all lower body movements.
- **Quadriceps** – This is the large group of muscles on the front of the upper leg, often referred to as the thighs. Their primary function is to flex the hip and extend the knee.
- **Hamstrings** – This is the group of muscles on the backside of the leg, running from the hip joint to the knee joint. Their primary function is to facilitate flexion of legs, medial and lateral rotation; important for walking, running and jumping.

## Back Squat

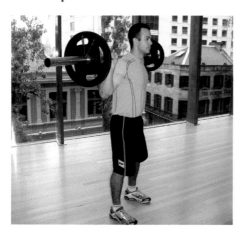

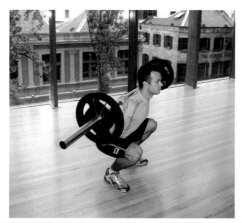

| Start | Midpoint |

### Instruction

- Stand with feet shoulder-width apart and bar resting across rear of shoulders with hands slightly wider than shoulder-width apart gripping bar.
- Maintaining the natural curve of your lower back, brace your stomach.
- Breathe in as you slowly bend at your knees, sit back and lower buttocks towards the ground to the appropriate angle – quarter, half or full squat.
- Keep your heels on the floor and resist leaning forward from the hips. Maintain ear over shoulder, over hip over ankle – from side position – and knees following the line of the toes.
- Breathe out as you raise body upwards using your legs to starting position.
- Maintain a continuous flowing movement at all times until repetitions are completed.

**Note:** This exercise can be performed lowering to a quarter squat, half-squat (90-degree leg angle) or full squat position.

# Front Squat

## Instruction

- Stand with feet shoulder-width apart and bar resting across front of shoulders with hands slightly wider than shoulder-width apart – elbows high, hands supporting (as shown).
- Maintaining the natural curve of your lower back, brace your stomach.
- Breathe in as you slowly bend at your knees, sit back and lower buttocks towards the ground to appropriate the angle – quarter, half or full squat
- Breathe out as you raise body upwards using your legs to starting position.
- Maintain a continuous flowing movement at all times until repetitions completed.

**Note:** This exercise can be performed lowering to a quarter squat, half-squat (90-degree leg angle) or full squat position. Practice wrist, forearm shoulder and back flexibility regularly to help keep elbows high at all times in order to perform this exercise correctly (see page 143-146).

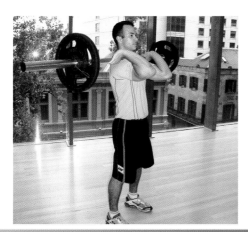 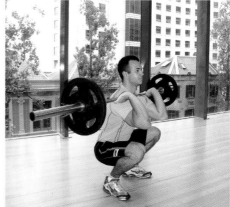

Start      Midpoint

## Stationary Leg Lunge

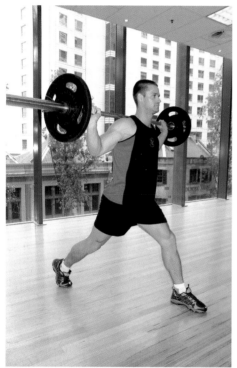 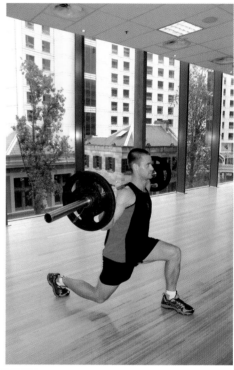

Start                                                    Midpoint

### Instruction

- Stand with your back straight, barbell across back of shoulders in forward lunge position with hands wider than shoulder-width apart – body raised.
- Maintaining the natural curve of your lower back, brace your stomach.
- Check that both your feet are facing forwards.
- Breathe in as you lower your rear knee towards the ground, though never touching.
- Breathe out and rise up.
- Ensure hips remain square at all times.
- Maintain a continuous flowing movement at all times until repetitions are completed, avoiding any arching of the lower back.
- Repeat drill with opposite leg forward.

**Note:** This exercise can also be performed with arms extended overhead. Also see Raised Lunge progression (page 119).

# Alternate Leg Lunge

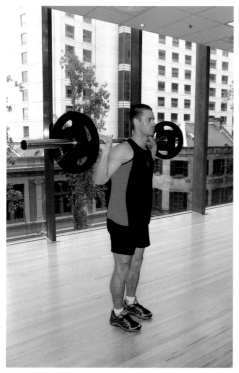 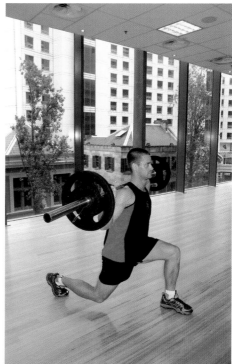

Start                                                    Midpoint

## Instruction

- Stand with your back straight, feet together, barbell across rear of shoulders with hands wider than shoulder-width gripping bar.
- Maintaining the natural curve of your lower back, brace your stomach.
- Breathe in as you take a lunge step forward with your left foot.
- Check that your feet are facing forward and your right knee is positioned on the midline of your toe and heel, lowering your right knee towards the ground, though never touching.
- Breathe out as you push firmly back, drawing your left leg back and stand upright. Push from your heel keeping your body tight.
- Ensure hips remain square at all times.
- Repeat lunging forward with opposite leg.
- Maintain a continuous flowing movement at all times until repetitions are completed.

**Note:** This exercise can also be performed with: (a) arms extended overhead (b) walking lunges – continually moving forwards.

## Leg Press

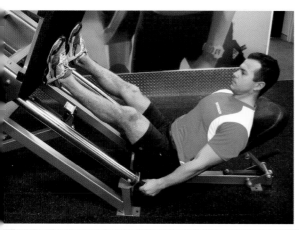 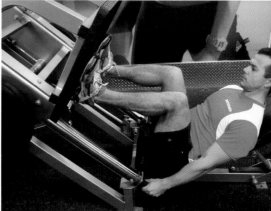

Start | Midpoint

### Instruction

- Sitting in leg press machine, position your feet shoulder-width apart against pressing board with toes pointed slightly outward.
- Grasp the handle grips or sides of the seat (machine specific).
- Breathing in, bend your knees as you lower the weight as far as possible bringing your knees towards your chest without changing the position of your hips. Avoid your hips lifting off the seat.
- Breathing out, push the weight back up using your heels, not your toes.
- Avoid locking your knees out at the top, but rather take the weight to just before.
- Maintain a continuous flowing movement at all times until repetitions are completed.

**Note:** Change your foot positions to vary the angle on the muscle being targeted.

# Single Leg Press

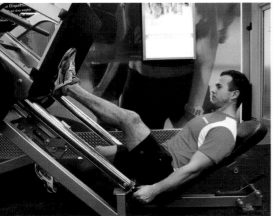

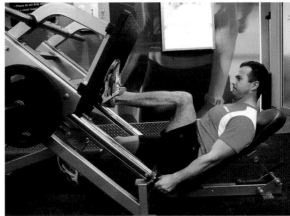

| Start | Midpoint |
|-------|----------|

## Instruction

- Sitting in leg press machine, position one foot in the center of the pressing board and the other leg lowered below.
- Grasp the handle grips or sides of the seat (machine specific).
- Breathing in, bend your knee as you lower the weight as far as possible bringing your knee towards your chest without changing the position of your hips. Avoid your hips lifting off the seat.
- Breathing out, push the weight back up using your heels, not your toes.
- Avoid locking your knees out at the top, but rather take the weight to just before.
- Maintain a continuous flowing movement at all times until repetitions completed.
- Repeat exercise on opposite leg.

**Note:** Change your foot positions to vary the angle on the muscle being targeted.

# Calves

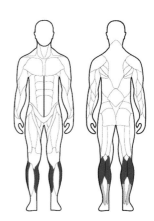

MUSCLE
WORKE

■ PRIMARY
Calves

■ SECONDA
Soleus

- **Calves** – The group of muscles on the back of the leg running from the backside of the knee to the Achilles tendon which bends the knee and points the toes (plantar flexion); helping us in walking, running, pedaling a bike and jumping.
- **Soleus** – The flat muscle underneath the calf muscle which acts only on the ankle joint to point the toes.

## Seated Calf Raise

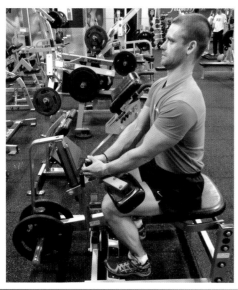
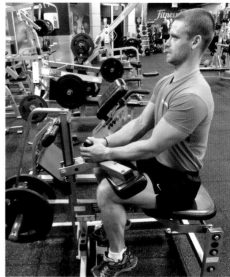

| Start | Midpoint |
|-------|----------|

### Instruction

- Sit in calf raise machine with your upper thighs resting against pads (adjust accordingly) and toes on edge of step lowering your heels.
- Breathing out, rise up onto your toes as high as possible and hold briefly.
- Breathe in and lower.

**Note:** Machines will vary in set-up positions. Alternatively, sit on edge of bench with weight resting on knees and raise and lower heels.

# Barbell Calf Raise – Rear

- Stand with feet shoulder-width apart and bar resting across rear of shoulders with hands slightly wider than shoulder-width apart gripping bar.
- Maintaining the natural curve of your lower back, brace your stomach.
- Breathing out, rise up onto your toes as high as possible and hold briefly.
- Breath-in and lower.
- Maintain a continuous flowing movement at all times until repetitions completed.

**Note:** This exercise can be performed using a stand up machine, but to assist with future Olympic lifting, this is a preferred method.

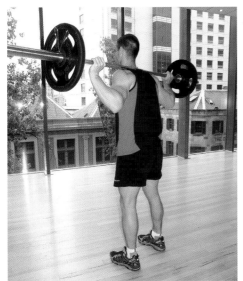 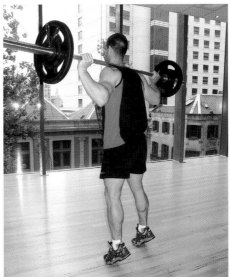

Start                                        Midpoint

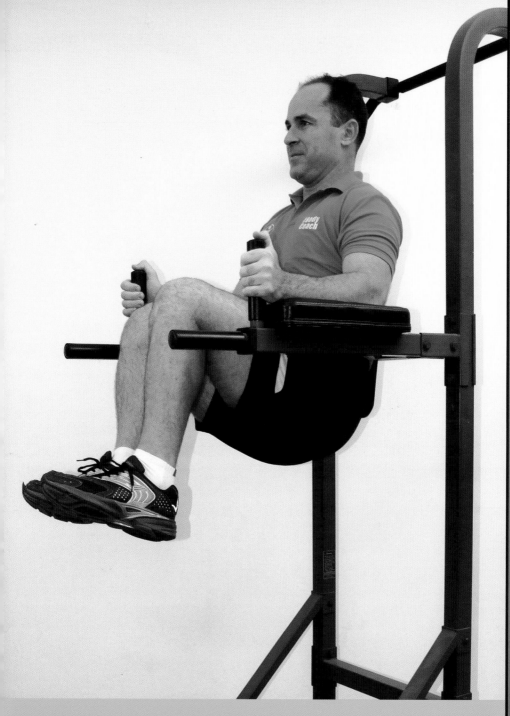

# Chapter 3

**Phase 2: Core Strength Development**

The abdominal and lower back muscles combine to form the core region of the body. The core region helps stabilize the body for more efficient and effective movement patterns to occur between the upper and lower body. Exercises that target the rectus abdominus and obliques work through various angles and intensities as well as the lower back and deeper transversus abdominus muscle. In addition, a number of compound exercises such as squats also strengthen the abdominal (torso) region.

# Core Abdominal, Obliques and Lower Back

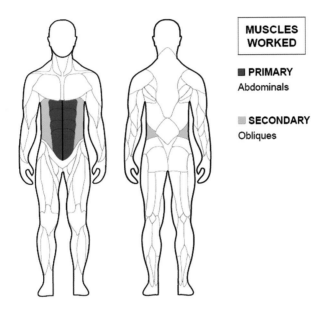

**MUSCLES WORKED**

■ **PRIMARY**
Abdominals

■ **SECONDARY**
Obliques

**Rectus Abdominus**
- Flexes the trunk.

**Obliques**
- Rotate, flex, bend trunk to the side. Support viscera and assist exhalation.

**Iliopsoas**
- Flexes the hips.

Abdominal exercises are often progressed through a series of core-isometric bracing and breathing drills to build static postural endurance. This is then followed by a series of muscular contraction exercises involving the abdominals and obliques as well as iliopsoas and lower back region, collectively referred to as the core region.

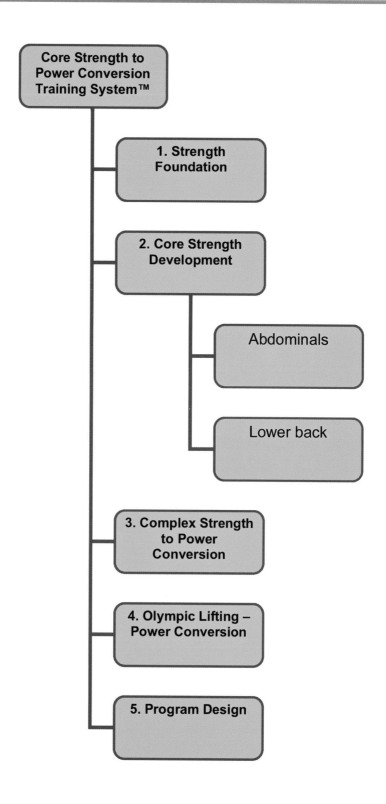

# Body Dish – Supine

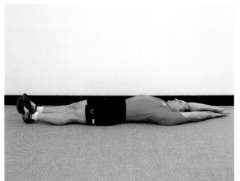 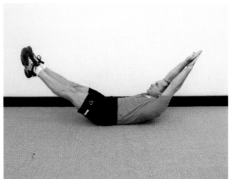

| Start | Raised |
|-------|--------|

## Instruction

- Lie in an extended position – legs together, toes pointed; arms overhead, hands together.

### 1. Dish Holds
- Simultaneously raise legs and arms into dish position and hold, ensuring deep breathing and strong abdominal brace is maintained for a set period of time (i.e. 5 or more seconds).

### 2. Repetition Based
- Lie in an extended position – legs together, toes pointed; arms overhead, hands together.
- Bracing your core abdominal region, contract musculature and simultaneously raise arms and legs into a body dish (banana) position, then lower maintaining long streamlined body position without relaxing.
- Repeat movement for set amount of repetitions with good form.
- Breathe out as you rise up (dish) and breathe in as you lower.

**Note:** To reduce the load, bend one leg and raise the other. Alternatively, place both hands on the thighs and slide hands towards knees as shoulders and legs rise off the ground.

## Medicine Ball Raise

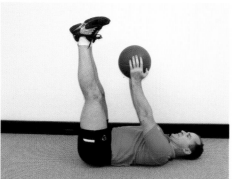 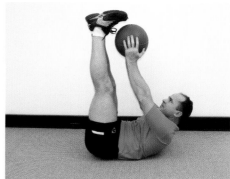

Start                                    Raised

### Instruction

- Lie on your back with legs raised from hip at 90 degrees and slightly bent.
- Extend arms up above eye line holding medicine ball.
- Breathing out, raise shoulders off the ground and reach medicine ball up towards feet, then lower.
- Avoid swinging legs or taking hip angle beyond 90 degrees due to the stress placed on the lower back region.
- Keep head neutral at all times. Avoid leading with chin, use abdominal muscles and maintain good form.

# Fitness Ball Abdominal Crunch

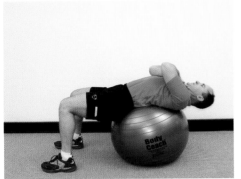

1. Hands across Chest

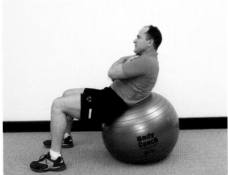

Level 1: Midpoint – Curl-up

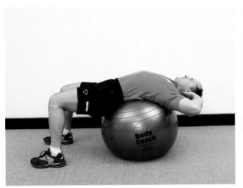

2. Hands behind Head

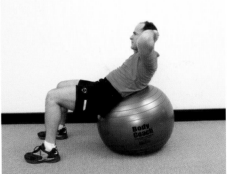

Level 2: Midpoint – Curl-up

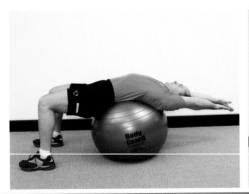

3. Arms Extended

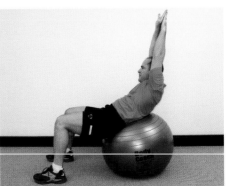

Level 3:  Midpoint – Curl-up

## Instruction

- Lie on fitness ball on arch of lower back, legs bent and feet shoulder-width apart.
- Level 1: Arms across chest
- Level 2: Hands behind head
- Level 3: Arms extended overhead

- Breathing out, contract the abdominal muscles and slowly crunch (curl) the stomach muscles up bringing the sternum towards the pelvis. Ensure the ball remains still whilst raising and lowering.
- Breathe in and lower.
- Raise and lower in a controlled manner to ensure tension in the abdominal muscles.
- Maintain the head in its neutral position throughout to avoid neck tension.

# Collins-Lateral Fly™ Series – Long Lever Holds

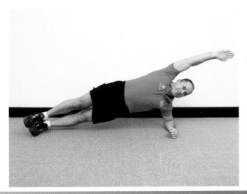 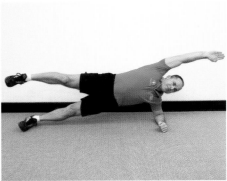

| 1. Raised Position | 2. Raise Leg |

## Instruction

- Lie on side with upper body supported by the elbow (90 degrees, directly below shoulder), forearm and clenched fist and lower body supported by feet – legs together.
- 1. Lift the pelvis off the ground, eliminating the side bending by raising up on the edge of shoes, forming a straight line from the feet to head – extending arm overhead.
- 2. Extend arm overhead and raise upper leg.
- Rise up and hold body position for three controlled breaths or 8-10 seconds – left side, then right side.

## Collins-Lateral Fly™ Series – Coordination Drills

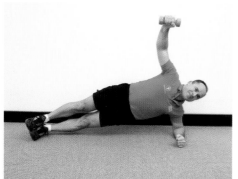

1. Start

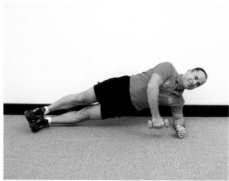

Lower and Raise Arm (Weighted)

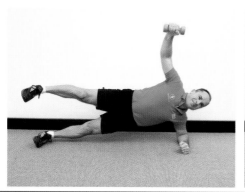

2. Raise Leg

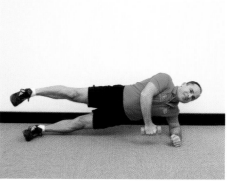

Lower and Raise Arm (Weighted) with Leg Raised

## Instruction

- Lie on side with upper body supported by the elbow, forearm and clenched fist. Lower body supported by feet – positioned together along with legs.
- Extend upper arm to open chest and raise into air.
- Lift the pelvis off the ground, eliminating the side bending by raising up on the edge of shoes, forming a straight line from the feet to head.
- Rise up and hold body position for three controlled breaths or 8-10 seconds whilst raising and lower arm. Repeat left side, then right side.
- 1. Lower and raise arm as a coordination drill in front of body.
- 2. Raise upper leg to increase the challenge whilst lowering and raising arm.
- Keep body tight – avoid any twisting or body rotation.

## Lateral Side Raises

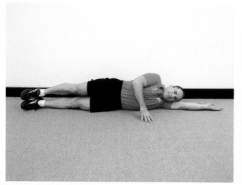 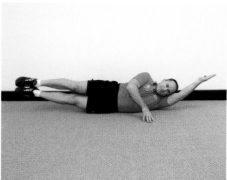

| Start | Midpoint – Legs and Arms Raised |

### Instruction

- Lie on your side, legs extended, toes pointed and feet together.
- The arm closest to the ground extends above head with palm facing towards ceiling – head relaxed resting on inner part of arm.
- The upper arm is bent, supporting your body weight in front of the body.
- Breathing in through the nose, then out through the mouth with pursed lips, draw your navel inwards and hold – maintaining a neutral spine.
- Maintaining a long body position, forcefully breathe out through pursed lips and simultaneously raise legs and arm into the air, then lower.
- Repeat on opposite side.
- This drill is performed rapidly.

**Note:** Maintain tight and long body position by leaning body slightly forward and putting weight onto hand supporting the body. Avoid leaning or falling backwards.

# Medicine Ball Elbow to Knee

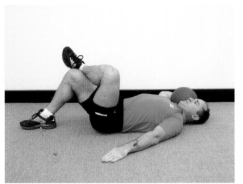
Start

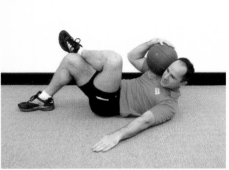
Elbow to Knee with Medicine Ball

## Instruction

- Lie on your back with one leg bent and the other foot resting on the opposite knee.
- Rest medicine ball on opposite shoulder to raised knee.
- Breathing out, raise opposite elbow towards opposite knee.
- Breathe in and lower.
- Repeat on opposite side.

## Lower Leg Lifts

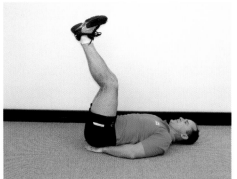 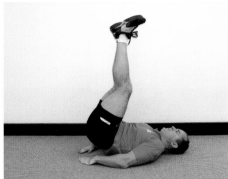

Start                                                    Raised

### Instruction

- Lie on your back with legs raised in the air and slightly bent and hands placed under your buttocks – palms down.
- Maintaining a strong abdominal brace, breathe out as you activate the lower abdominal region and raising the hip, legs and buttocks off the ground without swinging legs or changing their length.
- Breathe in as you lower buttocks to the ground in a controlled manner.

**Note:** Over time, with good abdominal contraction you will learn to relax the upper body and focus on solely activating the abdominal region.

# Knee Raise

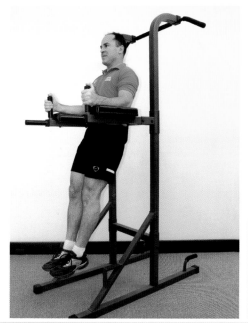 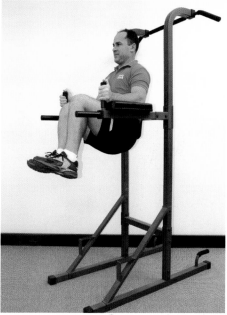

Start                                    Raised

## Instruction

- Position forearms on pads with shoulders kept high in Captain's Chair (or similar machine) with legs extended down and abdominal muscles braced.
- Maintain slight body dish position until exercise set is complete.
- Breathing out, raise knees to chest. Once thighs are parallel to ground, drive knees towards chest to obtain maximum abdominal contraction.
- Breath in and slowly lower legs to starting position.

**Note:** Avoid legs relaxing or swinging backwards when lowering.

## Hanging Knee Raises

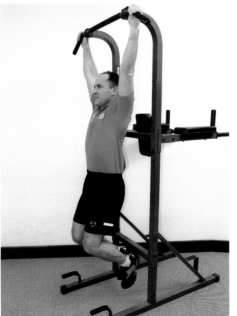 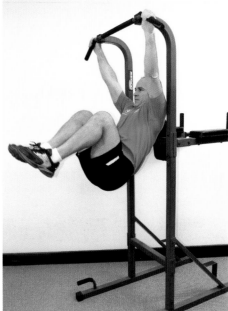

Start                                    Raised

### Instruction

- Grip an overhead bar with arms and legs extended and brace abdominal muscles.
- Breathing out, raise knees to chest, then lower legs slowly. Aim to maintain a tight body position at all times and avoid abdominal swinging (weakness).
- Breathe in and lower legs in a controlled movement.

**Note**: A coach may be necessary to support the lower back region of the participant to reduce swinging.

# Hip Raise – Shoulder Bridge

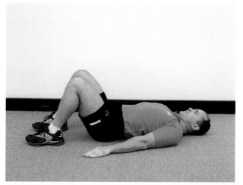 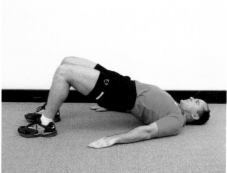

**Start**                                          **Midpoint – Raise Hips**

## Instruction

- Lie flat on back with legs bent and arms by your side.
- Breathe in deeply.
- Breathe out and slowly peel the lower back off the ground and raise hips into the air.
- Breathe in at the top of the movement and re-activate abdominal muscles and complete one full breath in and out.
- Breathe out and lower the body in reverse motion lowering hips to ground.

**Note:**
- Balance on heels and raise to introduce hamstrings muscle involvement.
- Maintain square hips at all times.
- To increase the intensity of the Hip Raise, extend one leg upwards and hold. Similar approach to resting on one heel to activate hamstrings muscles.

## Controlled Back Raise

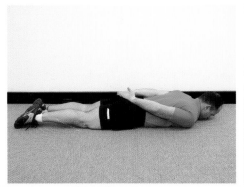
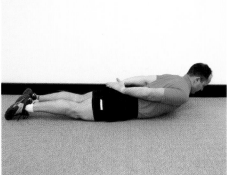

Start                                          Raised

### Instruction

- To strengthen the lower back region, lie on stomach with hands clasped behind back.
- Breathing out, contract stomach and raise upper body (chest) off floor.
- Focus on elongating the spine and rising away and up a short distance whilst maintaining braced abdominal muscles.
- Breathing in, slowly lower the chest back to the floor.

**Note**: No tension or pain should be felt in the lower back at any time during exercise. Stretch lower back in between sets by lying on your back and bringing your knees to your chest.

**Note:** For additional lower back exercise see page 54 for Back Raises exercise.

## Core Strength Workout

Core strength exercises can be performed on a daily basis. Exercises and specific regions can be rotated on a daily basis, for instance Abdominals Monday and Obliques Tuesday. As a coach I believe a higher number of repetitions are required for athletes than general strength training philosophy due to the lower intensity of each drill. In some instances, hundreds of repetitions are performed on the same drill for effective conditioning. Alternatively, time can be used to replace reps. As with all exercise, once the quality of movement fatigues, the exercise is stopped and recovery undertaken. Some exercises are performed slowly whilst others more rapidly. Refer to 8 Key Elements, page 19.

**Sample Workout 1:**

| EXERCISE | REPS | SETS | RECOVERY |
|---|---|---|---|
| 1. Body Dish | 15-30 | 3-5 | 60-seconds |
| 2. Lateral Side Raises | 20 | 3 sets each side | Nil. Move from one side onto the other |
| 3. Lower Leg Lifts | 15-30 | 3-5 | 60-seconds |
| 4. Controlled Back Raise | 8-15 | 3 | 60-seconds |
| Total volume | Up to 465 reps, depending on reps and sets | | |

**Sample Workout 2:**

| EXERCISE | REPS | SETS | RECOVERY |
|---|---|---|---|
| 1. Medicine Ball Raise | 15-30 | 3-5 | 60-seconds |
| 2. Medicine Ball Elbow to Knee | 20 | 3 sets each side | Nil. Move from one side onto the other |
| 3. Hanging Knee Raises | 10-20 | 3-5 | 60-90 seconds |
| 4. Hip Raise – Shoulder Bridge | 8-15 | 3 | 60-seconds |
| Total volume | Up to 415 reps, depending on reps and sets | | |

For additional core strength abdominal and lower back exercise see the following Body Coach Books including: Core Strength, Awesome Abs and Power Training.

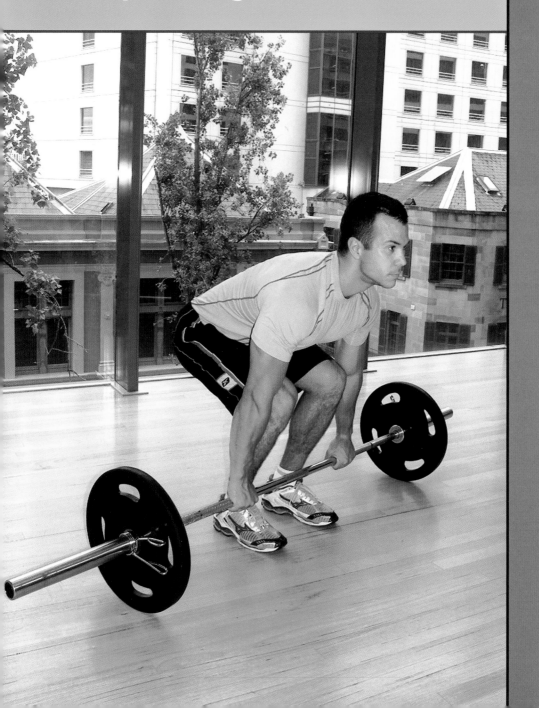

# Chapter 4

**Phase 3:**

**Complex Strength to Power Conversion**

Exercise progression plays an important role in developing strength and preparing the body for more advanced movement patterns. In foundation strength, the initial focus is based on very slow development of force (mass x acceleration) using both isolated and complex exercises that target specific muscle groups. The initial aim of this is towards increasing muscular size (or hypertrophy) before working through additional strength training cycles for maximal strength gains by increasing movement ratios. Combine this with the development of core strength in Phase 2 and the body will have established a great foundation working into this next phase of training.

Complex strength to power training provides a series of exercise progressions that help establish strength, speed, power and technique that ultimately leads into Olympic lifting power conversion. The exercise progressions are Olympic lifts broken down into a series of movement patterns that imitate specific phases of an Olympic lift. In this phase a rapid development of force contributes to the development of further speed and power whilst gradually acclimatizing the Central Nervous System (CNS) for additional demands, preparing the body for the higher demands of Olympic lifting itself.

As more complex exercises are introduced, you'll sense and feel a greater demand by the CNS in performing each exercise. The exercises themselves are becoming more functional and sports specific in many ways and have a much higher intensity. The strength gains from previous phases are now being placed through a conversion process where a higher power output is required, whilst at the same time establishing proper technique for the ultimate Olympic Lifting Power Conversion phase. Medicine ball training is also a great exercise tool to improve power output when working with athletes of all age groups as the mass is low but acceleration is rapid. For more details please refer to The Body Coach: Power Training Book.

## Exercise Progression and Technique

It is much easier to have an athlete learn the lifting progressions in order to coordinate, master and perform the movement pattern before you put it all together with more advanced Olympic lifts. This vital approach helps speed up the learning curve and makes certain that the athlete establishes good technique, neuromuscular coordination and power. This section is designed to ensure that you take the necessary steps in learning to perform the Clean Jerk and Snatch and their variations properly, as well as derive strength and power benefits from the movement progressions themselves.

Over the following chapter, I will take you through a series of exercise progressions based upon the Clean, Jerk and Snatch lifting patterns and their variations. These variations are used by athletes and gym-goers to optimize their strength, power and performance levels. The breakdown of exercises also provides a good option for athletes with limited range of movement or flexibility to still perform high intensity movements, such as a power clean instead of a competition Clean and Jerk.

Ultimately, the goal here is to gradually progress each athlete through a series of exercise progressions for explosive lifts that allow them to develop good technique and coordination by balancing strengths and weaknesses whilst participating in the rapid development of force that will contribute to the development of speed and power – Strength to Power Conversion. This phase is crucial in the overall outlook of training as it enables each participant to adapt and improve their knowledge and understanding for optimal training performance.

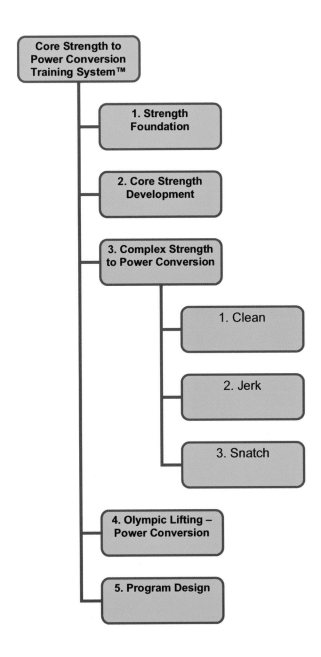

# 1. Clean

In this section are the progressive exercises used to teach athletes how to perform the Clean. Below is an example of the Clean being performed via a series of snapshots. On the following pages, the Clean has been broken down into 4 movement phases to assist in improving technique and initiating power conversion growth and development prior to attempting the more advanced competition lift, the Clean and Jerk.

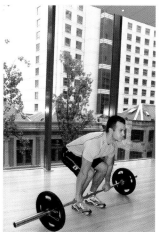

1. Start

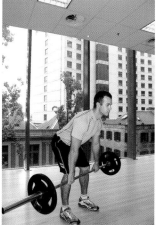

2. First Pull

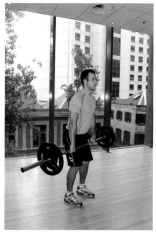

3. Scoop

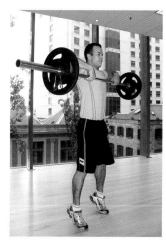

4. Second Pull

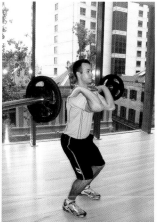

5. Descent Under Bar

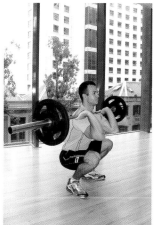

6. Catch

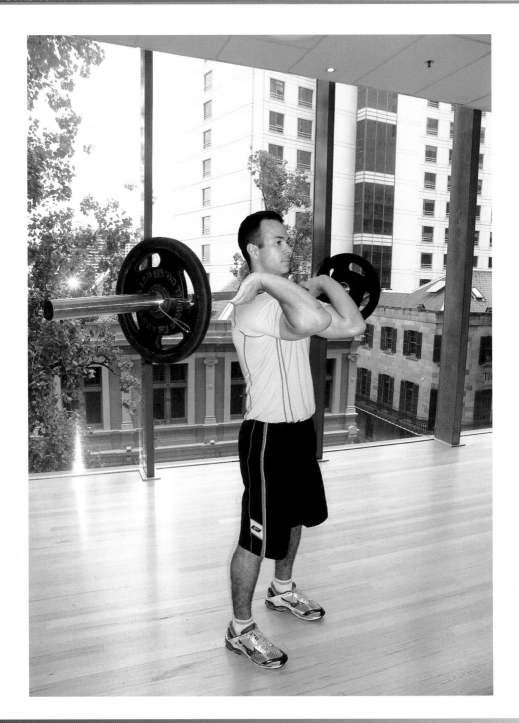

7. Finish

For full exercise instruction see Phase 4, page 147

# Clean – Phase 1

## Lift Phase

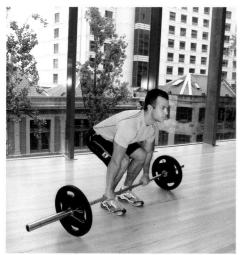 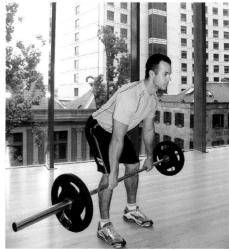

| Start | First Pull |

## Strength Specific – Exercise Breakdown Drills

### Dead-Lift (Page 56)

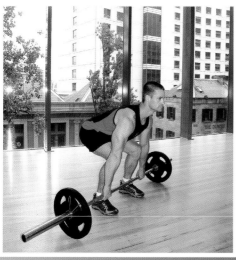 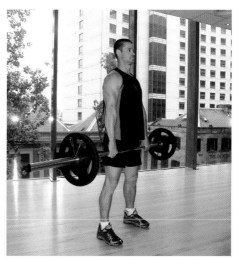

| Start | First Pull |

## Romanian Dead-Lift  (Page 53)

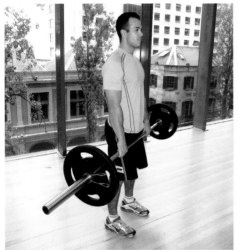 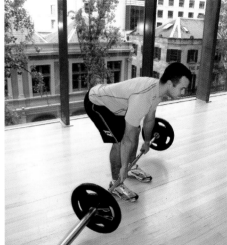

Start                                                    Midpoint

## Good Mornings (Page 55)

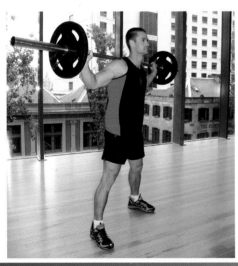 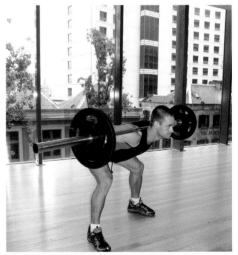

Start                                                    Midpoint

**Back Raises (Page 56)**

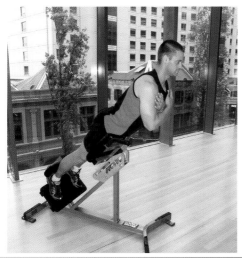

Start

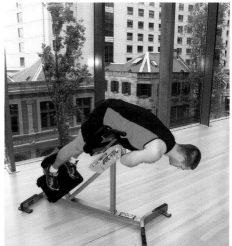

Midpoint

## Clean – Phase 2

### Scoop and Pull

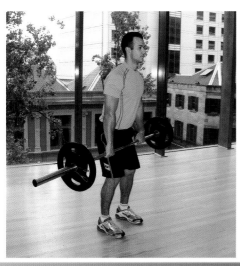

Scoop

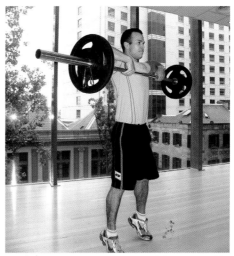

Second Pull

## Strength Specific – Exercise Breakdown Drills

### Calf Raises (Page 69)

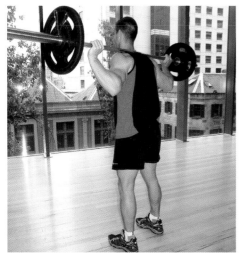 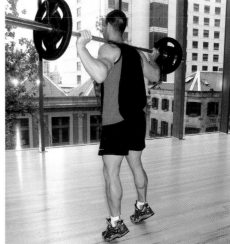

Start                                          Midpoint

### Bent Over Row (Page 49)

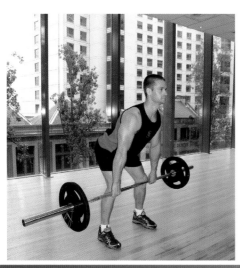 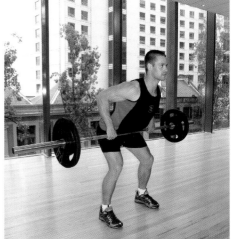

Start                                          Midpoint

**Upright Row - Close Grip   (Page 43)**

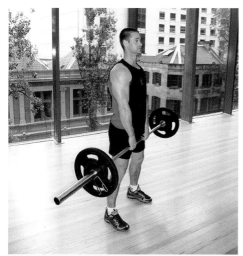

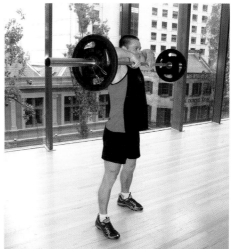

| Start | Midpoint |
|-------|----------|

**Upright Row – Wide Grip  (Page 43)**

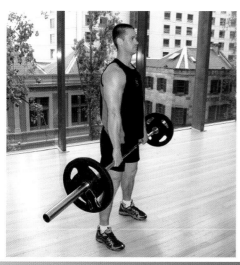

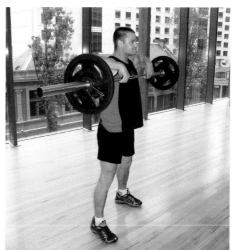

| Start | Midpoint |
|-------|----------|

**Shoulder Shrugs (Page 42)**

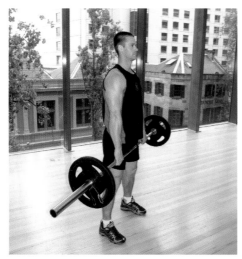

Start

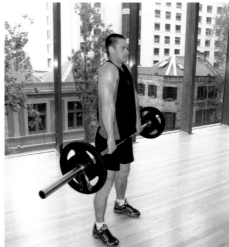

Midponit

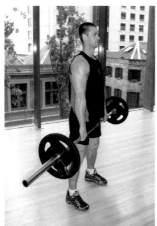

Start

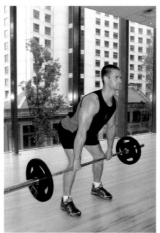

Lower

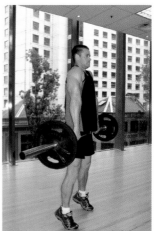

Power Up

## Hang Shrug

Stand with barbell in hands, feet at hip width, shoulders back and chest up. Keeping arms straight and eyes fixed forwards, lower the bar towards knees by moving the hips backward and establishing a slight bend in the knees. Breathing out quickly, move the hips forward as the hips extend explosively shrug shoulders and rise up on toes.

## Complex Exercise Progression – Drills

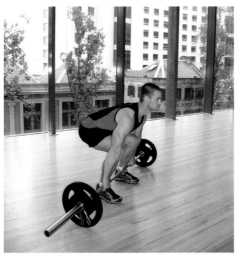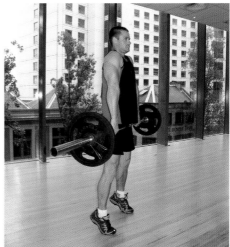

| Start | Upper Movement |

### Straight Arm Shrug

With barbell resting on ground, lower body into start position with feet approximately shoulder-width apart; shins close to the bar; knees and hips bent and arms extended holding bar slightly wider than shoulder-width outside knee alignment. Think hips, higher than knees but lower than shoulders – whilst arms are straight and extended down. Keeping arms straight and eyes fixed forwards, breathe out as you raise the bar up by driving with the legs. As the bar reaches towards the knees, quickly move the hips forward. As the hips extend explosively, shrug shoulders and rise up on toes, then lower.

**Hang High Pull**

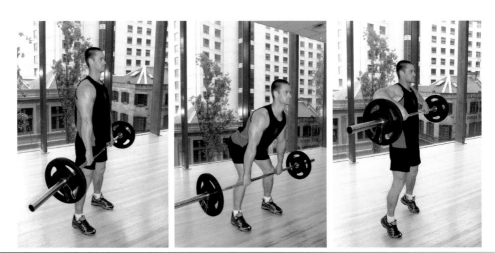

| Start | Lower | Power Up |

Stand with barbell in hands, feet at hip width, shoulders back and chest up. Keeping arms straight and eyes fixed forwards, raise the bar by moving the hips backwards while maintaining a slight but fixed bend in the knees. Stop once the bar reaches the top of the knees or when the flexibility in the hams runs out. Quickly move the hips forward, as the hips extend, explosively shrug shoulders and rise onto toes. Continue to elevate the bar to mid-chest height by bending elbows and continuing the upward movement of the bar. Be sure to lift elbows up and keep the bar close to the body. Control bar at completion of movement when lowering, keeping body tight.

## High Pull

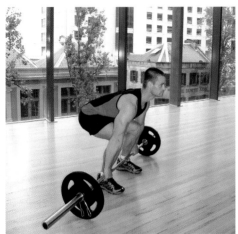
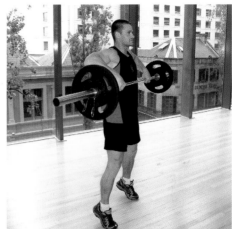

| Start | Upper Movement |
|-------|----------------|

With barbell resting on ground, lower body into start position with feet approximately shoulder-width apart; shins close to the bar; knees and hip bent and arms extended holding bar slightly wider than shoulder-width outside knee alignment. Think hips, higher than knees but lower than shoulders – whilst arms are straight and extended down. Keeping arms straight and eyes fixed forwards, breathe out as you raise the bar up by driving with the legs. As the bar reaches towards the knees, quickly move the hips forward. As the hips extend explosively, shrug shoulders and rise up on toes. Continue to elevate the bar to mid-chest height by bending elbows and continuing the upward movement of the bar. Be sure to lift elbows up and keep the bar close to the body. Control bar at completion of movement when lowering, keeping body tight.

# Clean – Phase 3

## Descent Under Bar and Finish

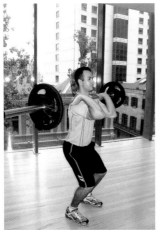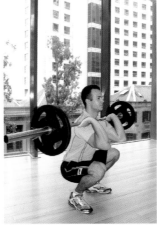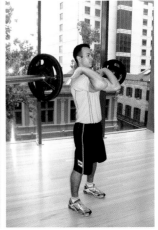

| 4. Descent Under Bar | 5. Catch | 6. Finish |

## Strength Specific – Exercise Breakdown Drills

### Back Squat – Variations (Page 62)
Quarter Squat; Half Squat; Full Squat

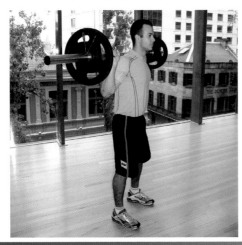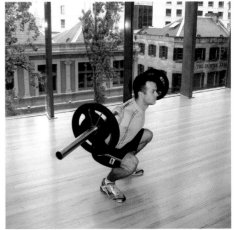

| Start | Midpoint |

## Front Squat Variations (Page 62)
Quarter Squat; Half Squat; Full Squat

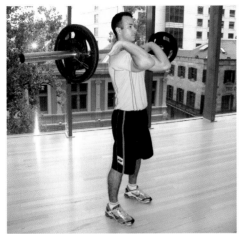 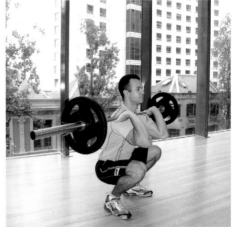

Start                                                    Midpoint

## Complex Exercise Progression – Drills

### Hang Power Cleans

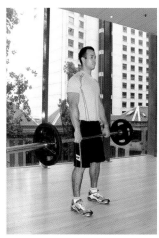 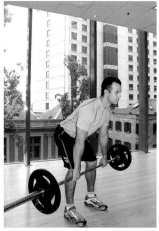 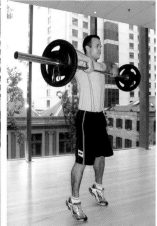

| Start | Lower | Pull |

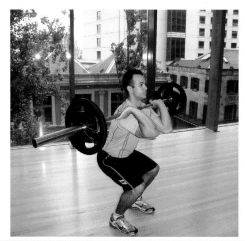 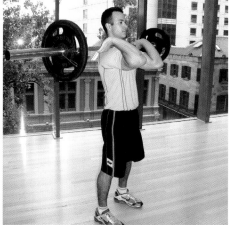

| Descent under Bar | Finish |

Stand with barbell in hand, feet at shoulder width, shoulders back and chest up. Keeping arms straight and eyes fixed forwards, raise the bar by moving the hips backwards and slightly bend the knees. As the bar lowers towards the knees, quickly move the hips forward. As the hips extend, explosively shrug the shoulders and rise up on toes. Continue to elevate the bar to mid-chest height by bending elbows and continuing the upward movement of the bar – kept close to the body. Once at shoulder height, simultaneously rotate elbows underneath the bar, releasing the grip and allowing the bar to fall onto the shelf created by the shoulders while lowering into a quarter squat – reached at the same time the barbell is received on the shoulders – before rising to standing position.

# Complex Exercise Progression - Drills

## Hang Cleans

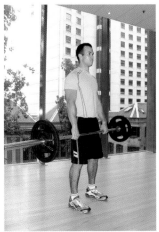
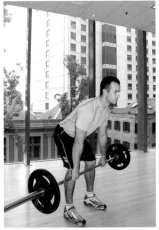
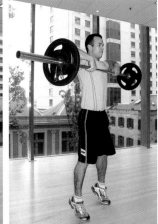

| Start | Lower | Power Up |

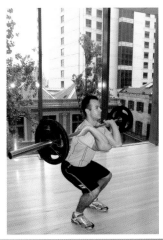
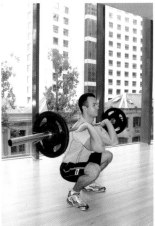
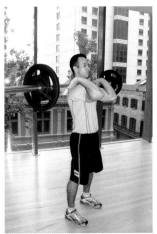

| Descent under Bar | Catch | Finish |

Stand with barbell in hand, feet at shoulder width, shoulders back and chest up. Keeping arms straight and eyes fixed forwards raise the bar by moving the hips backwards and slight bend in the knees. As the bar lowers towards the knees, quickly move the hips forward. As the hips extend explosively, shrug the shoulders and rise up on toes. Continue to elevate the bar to mid-chest height by bending elbows and continuing the upward movement of the bar – kept close to the body. Once at shoulder height, simultaneously rotate elbows underneath the bar, releasing the grip and allowing the bar to fall onto the shelf created by the shoulders while lowering into a full squat – reached at the same time the barbell is received on the shoulders, before rising to standing position.

# Complex Exercise Progression – Drills

## Muscle Cleans

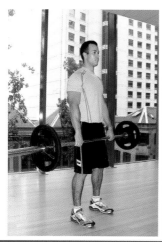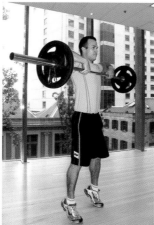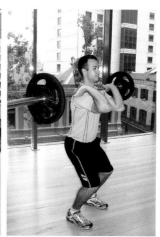

Standing tall with barbell in hands in clean grip and feet shoulder-width apart, breathe out as you slide bar upwards almost along the body to near shoulder height. Once at shoulder height, rotate elbows underneath the bar, releasing the grip and allowing the bar to fall onto the shelf created by the shoulders and catching with slightly bent knees before rising.

# Clean – Phase 4 (Power Clean)

### Complex Exercise Progression – Drills

To effectively perform the Power Clean, a modified version of the Clean, the athlete must lift the weighted bar from the ground to the chest and shoulders in one continuous movement as shown below

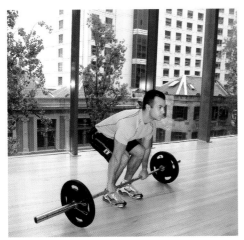

1. Start

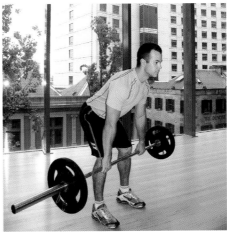

2. First Pull

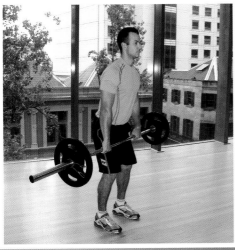

3. Scoop

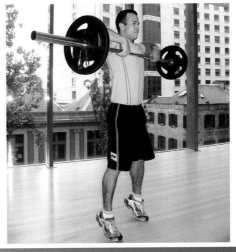

4. Second Pull

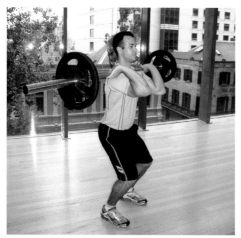 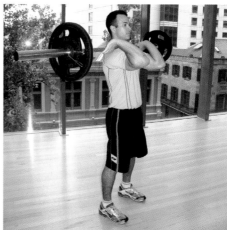

5. Descent Under Bar          6. Finish

With barbell resting on ground, lower body into start position with feet approximately shoulder-width apart; shins close to the bar; knees and hips bent and arms extended, holding bar slightly wider than shoulder width outside knee alignment. Think hips, higher than knees but lower than shoulders – whilst arms are straight and extended down. Keeping arms straight and eyes fixed forwards breathe out as you raise the bar up by driving with the legs. As the bar reaches towards the knees, quickly move the hips forward. As the hips extend explosively, shrug shoulders and rise up on toes. Continue to elevate the bar to mid-chest height by bending elbows and continuing the upward movement of the bar. Be sure to lift elbows up and keep the bar close to the body. Once near shoulder height, simultaneously rotate elbows underneath the bar, releasing the hook grip and letting the bar fall onto the shelf created by the shoulders while lowering the legs into a quarter squat position, before rising. The depth of the drop ultimately depends on the height of the pull. In saying this, the squat should be reached at the same time the barbell is received on the shoulders.

# 2. Jerk

In this section are the progressive exercises used to teach athletes how to perform the Jerk. Below is an example of the Jerk being performed via a series of snapshots. On the following pages, the Jerk has been broken down into 3 movement phases to assist in improving technique and initiating power conversion growth and development prior to attempting the more advanced competition lift – the Clean and Jerk.

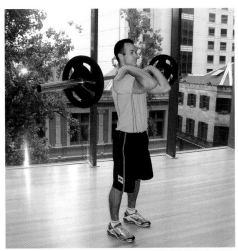
1. Start Position

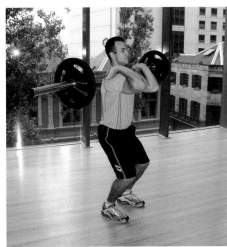
2. Knee and Hip Flexion

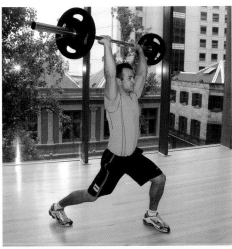
3. Extend and Catch

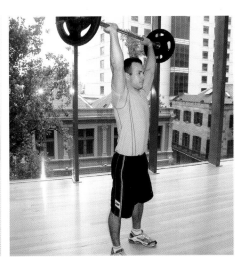
4. Front Foot Recovery and Finish Position

For full exercise instruction see Phase 4, page 147-149 (Clean and Jerk)

## Jerk Phase 1

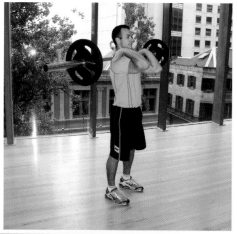 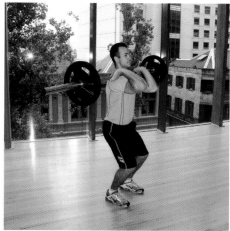

| 1. Start Position | 2. Knee and Hip Flexion |

## Strength Specific – Exercise Breakdown Drills

### Back Squat – Variations (Page 62)

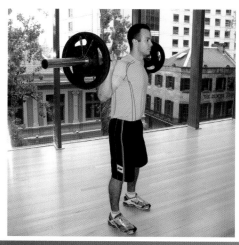 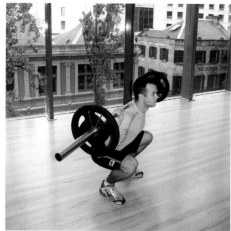

| 1. Start Position | 2. Knee and Hip Flexion |

- Quarter Squat
- Half Squat
- Full Squat

## Front Squat Variations (Page 63)

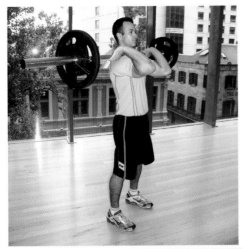 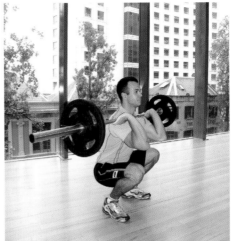

| 1. Start Position | 2. Knee and Hip Flexion |

- Quarter Squat
- Half Squat
- Full Squat

## Jerk Phase 2

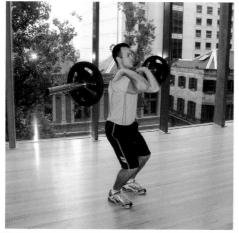

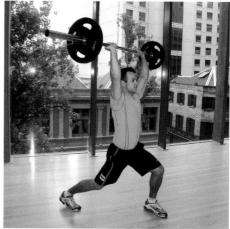

2. Knee and Hip Flexion

3. Extend and Catch

## Strength Specific – Exercise Breakdown Drills

**Shoulder Press – Rear  (Page 49)**

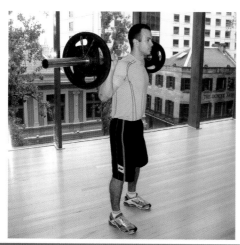

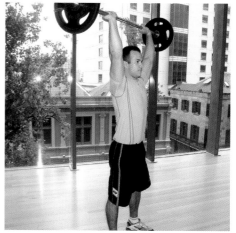

Start

Midpoint

## Shoulder Press – Front (Page 40)

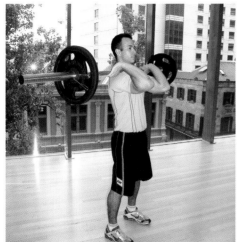 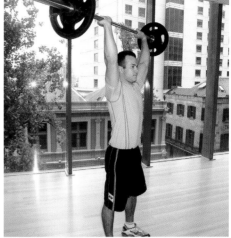

Start                                 Midpoint

## Stationary Lunge (Page 64)

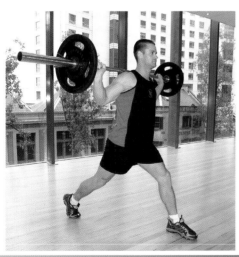 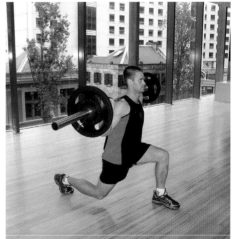

Start                                 Midpoint

**Alternate Leg Lunge (Page 65)**

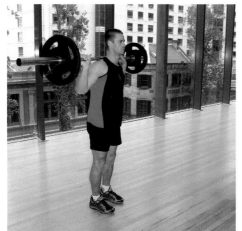 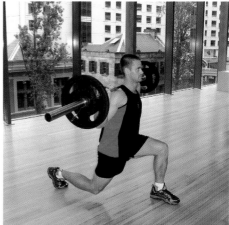

Start                                                    Midpoint

# Complex Exercise Progression – Drills

## Barbell Push Press – Front

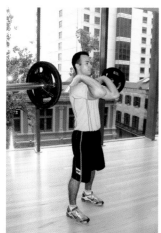 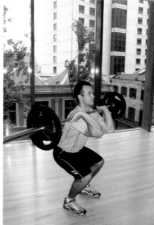 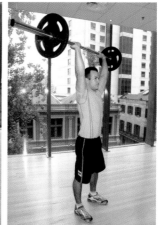

| Start | Lower | Raise |

Start with barbell resting on front of shoulders and support with hands at shoulder width – keeping the elbows high. Breathing in, drop the hips slightly as part of the initial movement before breathing out and exploding up. The objective is to aggressively push up on the bar after driving the legs. Unlike the military press, the athlete should not be using the arms to drive the weight, but instead use the hips and legs. The Push Press exercise is used to improve jerk drive through the use of the legs as the primary mover.

## Push Jerk – Semi Squat

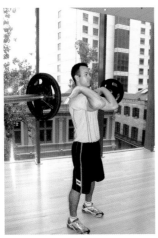 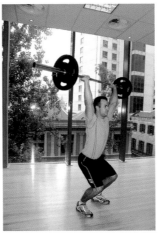 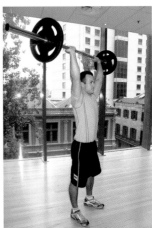

| Start | Dip | Raise |

Start with barbell resting on front of shoulders and support with hands at shoulder width – keeping the elbows high. Breathing out, simultaneously dip, keeping the torso rigid and vertical with the weight positioned through the center of the feet. Thrust up explosively onto the toes then rapidly dip under the bar into a semi-squat position – locking the arms and bar above the head before standing up.

**Note:** A similar movement may be performed with bar resting behind the neck.

## Push Jerk – Deep Squat

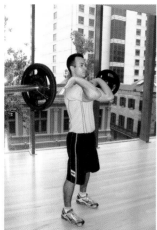 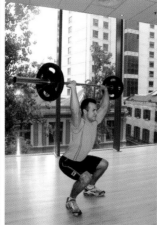 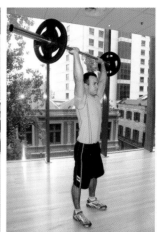

| Start | Dip | Raise |

Start with barbell resting on front of shoulders and support with hands at shoulder width – keeping the elbows high. Breathing out, simultaneously dip, keeping the torso rigid and vertical with the weight through the center of the feet, before thrusting up explosively onto the toes then rapidly dip under the bar into a near full-squat position – locking the arms and bar above the head before standing up.

**Note:** A similar movement may be performed with bar resting behind the neck.

## Split Jerk

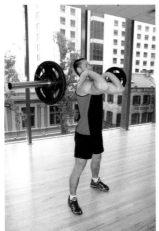 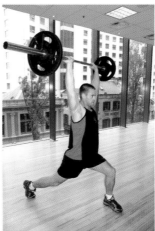 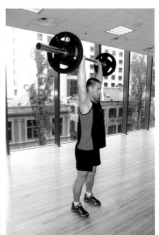

| Start | Jump | Raise |

Start with barbell resting on front of shoulders and support with hands at shoulder width – keeping the elbows high. Breathing out, simultaneously dip, and jump into forward lunge position whilst rapidly driving arms up overhead.

Keep underneath the bar while moving one foot forward and the other back. The thigh of the front leg should be roughly parallel to the floor, and the rear foot should be on the toes, with a small bend in the leg. Step forwards and bring feet close together, hold briefly before lowering bar.

# Jerk Phase 3

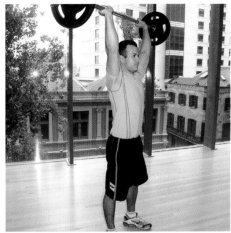 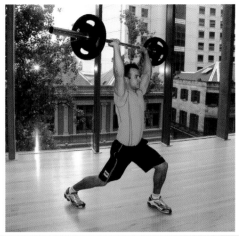

| 3. Extend and Catch | 4. Front Foot and Finish Position |

## Strength Specific – Exercise Breakdown Drills

### Raised Lunge

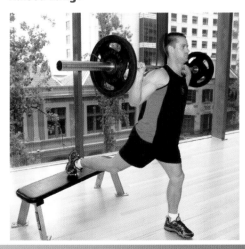 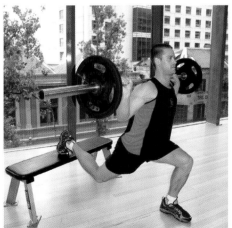

| Start | Midpoint |

Stand tall with barbell resting on rear of shoulders and hands slightly wider than shoulder width. Extend one leg back up onto flat bench positioned two steps behind. Breathe in and lower rear knee towards ground – keeping pelvis square and avoiding arching of the lower back at all times. Breathe out and rise up again. Repeat with opposite leg.

**Note:** Ensure that a strong and stable commercial bench is used on a non-slip surface.

## Overhead Stationary Lunge

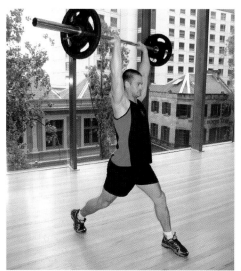 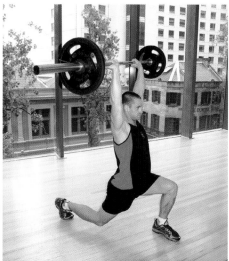

Start                                    Midpoint

Stand tall in forward lunge position with arms extended overhead holding dumbbell. Breathe in and lower rear knee towards ground – keeping pelvis square and avoiding arching of the lower back at all times. Breathe out and rise up again. Repeat with opposite leg forward.

# Complex Exercise Progression – Drills

## Step Ups

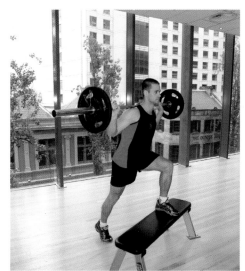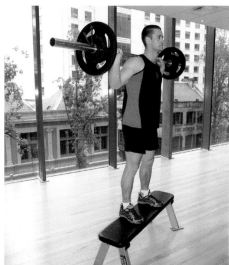

Start                                                        Midpoint

Stand tall behind flat bench with barbell resting on rear of shoulders and hands slightly wider than shoulder-width apart. Tighten your stomach muscles to support your lower back. Leading with your left leg, breathe out as you step up onto the bench and then follow with the right leg. Once standing upon bench with both feet, lower your feet back to the starting position leading with your left leg. Repeat movement starting with your right leg.

**Note:** Ensure that a strong and stable commercial bench is used on a non-slip surface.

### Forward Lunge to Press

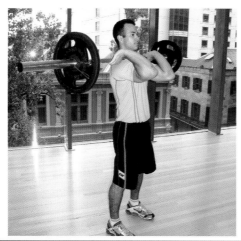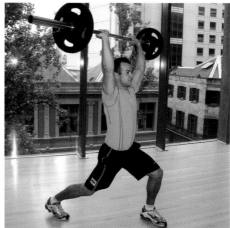

Start | Lunge Press

Start with barbell resting on front of shoulders and support with hands at shoulder width – keeping the elbows high. Breathing out, simultaneously step forward into lunge position whilst rapidly driving arms up overhead. Keep underneath the bar while moving one foot forwards. Step forwards before lowering bar and repeating with opposite leg.

### Hang Clean and Jerk
This exercise combines phases of the clean and the jerk from a hang position.

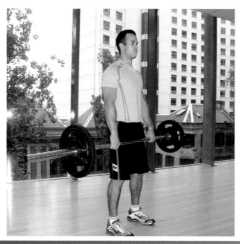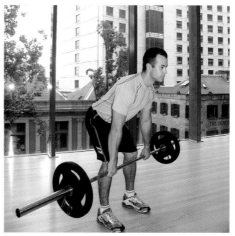

1. Start Position | 2. Lower Forwards

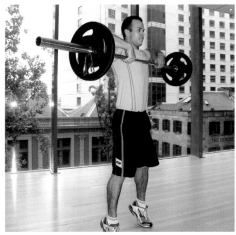

3. Pull

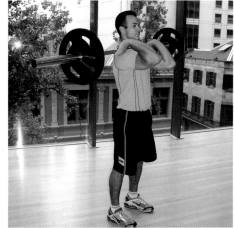

4. Scoop

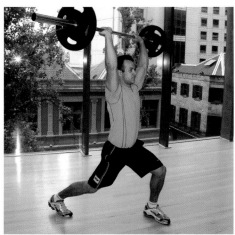

5. Extend and Catch

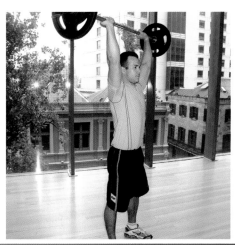

6. Front Foot and Finish Position

# 3. Competition Snatch

In this section are the progressive exercises used to teach athletes how to perform the Snatch. Below is an example of the Snatch being performed via a series of snapshots. On the following pages, the Snatch has been broken down into 4 movement phases to assist in improving technique and initiating power conversion growth and development prior to attempting the more advanced Competition Snatch exercise.

**There are two major elements found in the Snatch exercise including:**

1. Wide hand grip – Raise arms up parallel to ground. Bend elbows at 90-degrees with fingers pointing down. Lower down to bar by bending legs. Grip bar in this position, then straighten arms for wide grip position.

2. Hook hand grip on bar – This entails holding the thumb with the index and forefingers once the bar has been grasped. (see page 29)

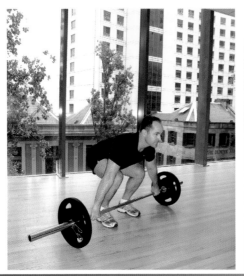 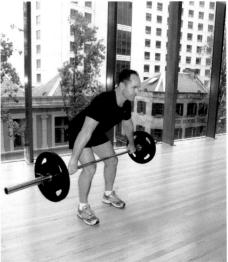

| 1. Start Position | 2. First Pull |

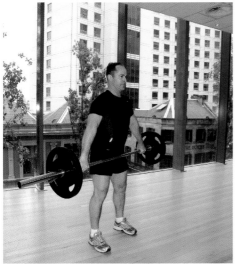

3. Scoop

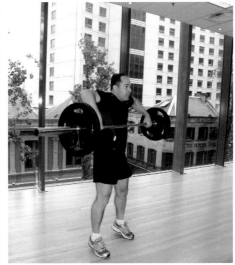

4. Second Pull

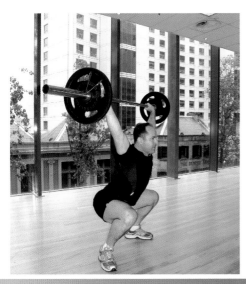

5. Descent under Bar & Catch

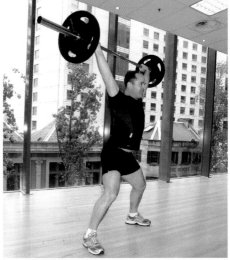

6. Finish

For full exercise instruction see Phase 4, page 152.

## Competition Snatch – Phase 1

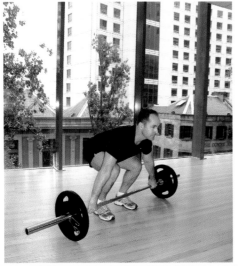 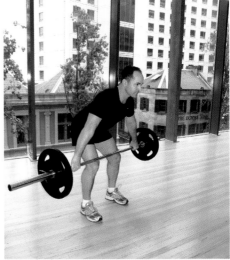

Start Position                          2. First Pull

## Strength Specific –
Exercise Breakdown Drills

### Snatch Grip Dead-Lift (Page 124)

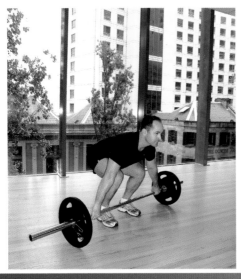 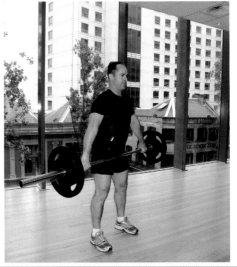

Start                                   Midpoint

## Good Mornings (Page 55)

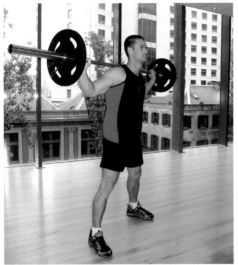 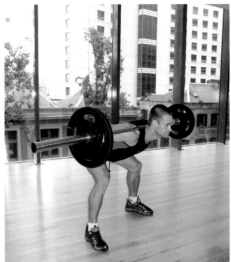

Start                                    Midpoint

## Competition Snatch – Phase 2

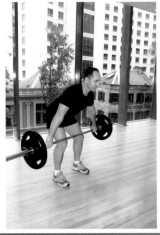
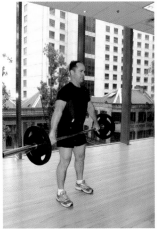
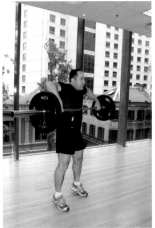

2. First Pull       3. Scoop       4. Second Pull

## Strength Specific – Exercise Breakdown Drills

**Bent Over Row (Page 49)**

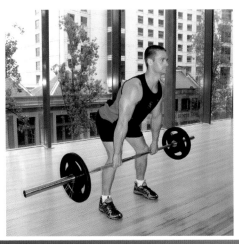
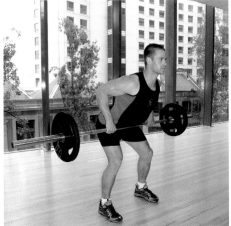

Start       Midpoint

## Upright Row – Snatch Grip (Page 43)

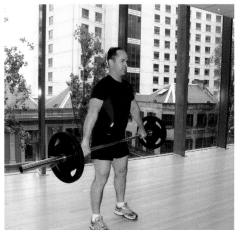 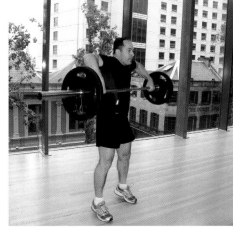

Start                                    Midpoint

## Complex Exercise Progression – Drills

### Snatch Hang Pull

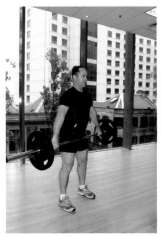 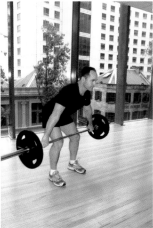 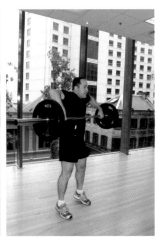

| Start | Lower | Pull |

Stand with the barbell in your hands with a hook grip, feet at shoulder width, shoulders back and chest up and over the bar. Keeping arms straight and eyes fixed forwards, initially lower bar by moving the hips backward while maintaining a slight but fixed bend in the knees with shoulders forwards. As the bar reaches the top of the knees, rapidly return to the starting position by driving the hips forward and standing up straight – driving up onto the toes. Once you are up on the toes, continue to elevate the bar to mid-chest height by bending the elbows and continuing the upward movement of the bar. Be sure to lift elbows up and keep the bar close to the body.

## Snatch Shrug

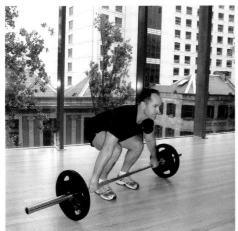 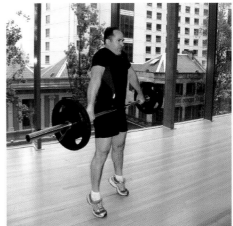

Start                                                      Drive-up

Stand over the bar with the balls of the feet positioned under the bar shoulder-width apart. Squat down and grip bar with hook grip, arms straight and elbows pointed along the bar. Pull the bar up off the ground by extending the hips and knees, keeping the bar as close to the legs as possible. As you raise the bar up to the knees, the torso still maintains the same angle to the floor as in the starting position, before driving the hips forward and standing up straight as the bar passes onto the thighs – driving up onto the toes, vigorously raising the shoulders up whilst keeping the arms straight.

**Snatch Pull**

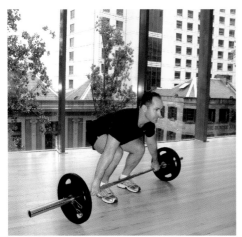 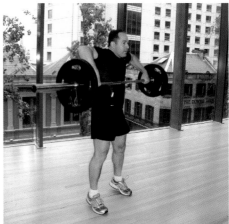

Start                                                    Drive-up

Stand over the bar with the balls of the feet positioned under the bar shoulder-width apart. Squat down and grip bar with hook grip, arms straight and elbows pointed along the bar. Pull the bar up off the ground by extending the hips and knees, keeping the bar as close to the legs as possible. As you raise the bar up to the knees, the torso still maintains the same angle to the floor as in the starting position, before driving the hips forward and standing up straight as the bar passes onto the thighs – driving up onto the toes. Once you are up on the toes, continue to elevate the bar to mid-chest height by bending elbows and continuing the upward movement of the bar. Be sure to lift elbows up and keep the bar close to the body.

# Competition Snatch – Phase 3

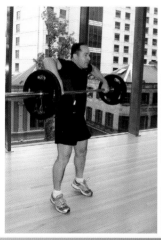 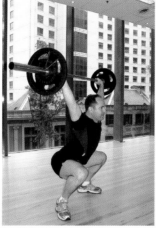 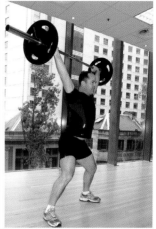

| 4. Second Pull | 5. Descent under Bar & Catch | 6. Finish Position |

## Strength Specific –
Exercise Breakdown Drills

### Overhead Squat

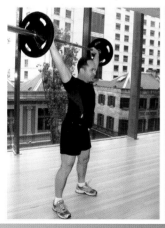 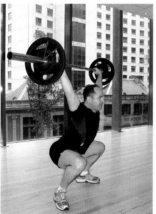 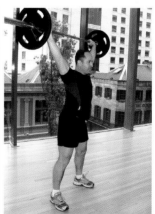

| Start | Midpoint | End Point |

Start with bar overhead with snatch hook grip and feet wider than shoulder width. Breathe in as you lower body towards the floor by bending the knees into a squat position. The arms are maintained over and behind head alignment with the weight over mid-feet for good center of gravity. Upon reaching end position, breathe out whilst rising to start position.

**Note:** This is an advanced exercise that requires focus on both upper and lower body flexibility and core strength. Practice first using the bar only under the guidance of a Strength and Conditioning Coach to ensure correct technique is obtained.

## Complex Exercise Progression – Drills

### Press Behind Neck – Snatch Grip

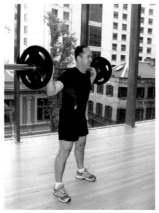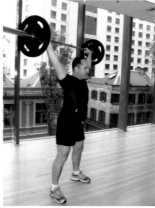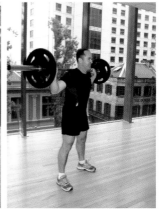

| Start | Raise | Lower |

Rest bar bend neck across shoulders with arms and hands in snatch position with hook grip. Maintain neutral spine position and brace stomach. Breathe out and extend arms overhead. Breathe in and lower bar.

### Push Press (Rear) – Wide Grip

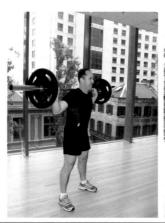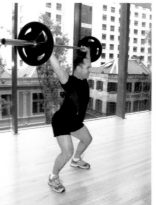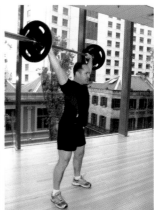

| Start | Press | Finish |

Rest bar bend neck across shoulders with arms and hands in snatch position with hook grip. Maintain neutral spine position and brace stomach. Breathe in and slightly bend knees before rapidly exploding legs up whilst breathing out and allowing momentum of leg drive to push bar up overhead. Briefly hold bar overhead before lowering.

## Pressing Snatch Balance

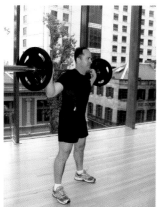 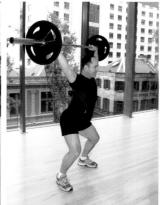 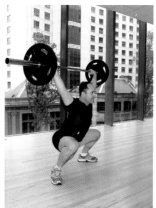

| Start | Press | Lower |

Rest bar bend neck across shoulders with arms and hands in snatch position with hook grip. Maintain neutral spine position and brace stomach. Breathe out as you simultaneously bend knees and lower body under bar into overhead squat position whilst raising bar up overhead.

## Drop Snatch

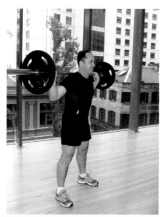 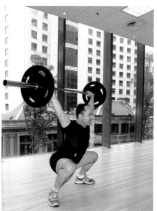 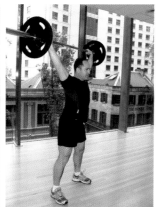

| Start | Drop | Raise |

Rest bar bend neck across shoulders with arms and hands in snatch position with hook grip. Maintain neutral spine position and brace stomach. Breathe in as you take a small dip down, then extend the legs and as soon as the bar leaves the shoulders, rapidly lower into a full squat position whilst locking the arms out with the bar overhead and breathing out. Raise back up straightening legs and lower bar to shoulders.

## Hang Power Snatch

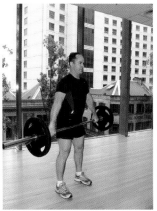 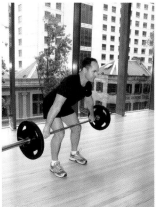 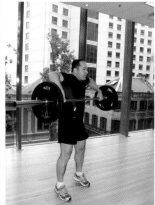

| Start | Lower | Pull |

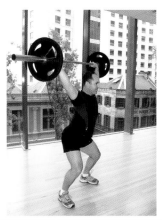 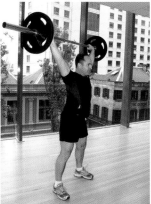

| Descent | Finish |

Stand with the barbell in snatch position with hook grip, feet at shoulder width, shoulders back and chest up and over the bar. Keeping arms straight and eyes fixed forwards, initially lower bar by moving the hips backward while maintaining a slight but fixed bend in the knees and shoulders forward. As the bar reaches the top of the knees, rapidly return to the starting position by driving the hips forward and standing up straight – driving up onto the toes. Continue to elevate the bar to mid-chest height and beyond by bending the elbows and continuing the upward movement of the bar whilst dipping the body under into a semi-squat position. As the momentum carries the bar overhead and the arms lock out, straighten the legs to finish the movement. Be sure to keep the bar close to the body at all times.

## Hang Snatch to Overhead Squat

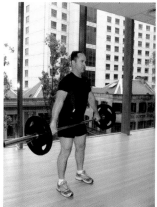

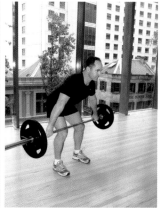

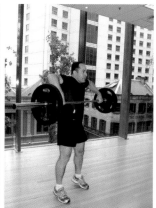

| Start | Lower | Pull |

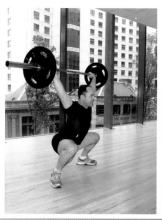

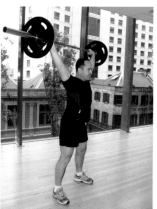

| Descent and Squat | Finish |

Stand with the barbell in your hands with a hook grip, feet at shoulder width, shoulders back and chest up and over the bar. Keeping arms straight and eyes fixed forwards, initially lower bar by moving the hips backwards while maintaining a slight but fixed bend in the knees and shoulders forwards. As the bar reaches the top of the knees, rapidly return to the starting position by driving the hips forward and standing up straight – driving up onto the toes; elevating the bar to mid-chest height and beyond by bending the elbows and continuing the upward movement of the bar whilst rapidly dipping the body under into a deep squat position. As the momentum of the drive carries the bar overhead, lock the arms out straight as you reach full squat position, before rising into a standing position with bar remaining overhead. Be sure to keep the bar close to the body at all times.

## Power Snatch – Phase 4

### Complex Exercise Progression – Drills

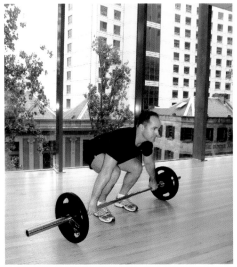

1. Start Position

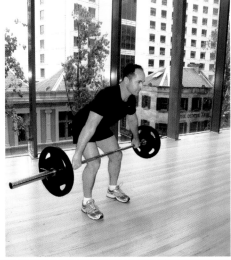

2. First Pull

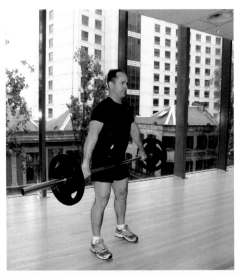

3. Scoop

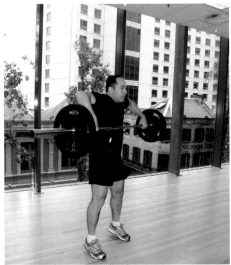

4. Second Pull

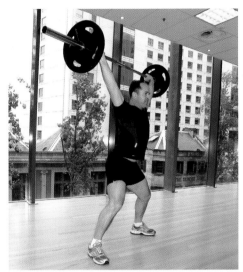 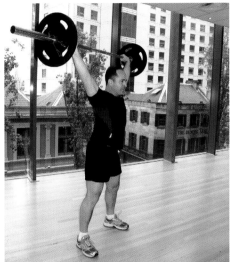

**Descent under Bar and Catch**                    **Finish Position**

Stand over the bar with the balls of the feet positioned under the bar shoulder-width apart. Squat down and grip bar with hook grip, arms straight and elbows pointed along the bar.

Pull the bar up off the ground by extending the hips and knees, keeping the bar as close to the legs as possible. As you raise the bar to the knees, the torso still maintains the same angle to the floor as in the starting position, before driving the hips forward and standing up straight as the bar passes onto the thighs – driving up onto the toes. Continue to elevate the bar to mid-chest height and beyond by bending the elbows and continuing the upward movement of the bar whilst dipping the body under into a semi-squat position. As the momentum carries the bar overhead and the arms lock out, straighten the legs to finish the movement. Be sure to keep the bar close to the body at all times.

# Chapter 5

**Phase 4:**

**Olympic Lifting – Power Conversion**

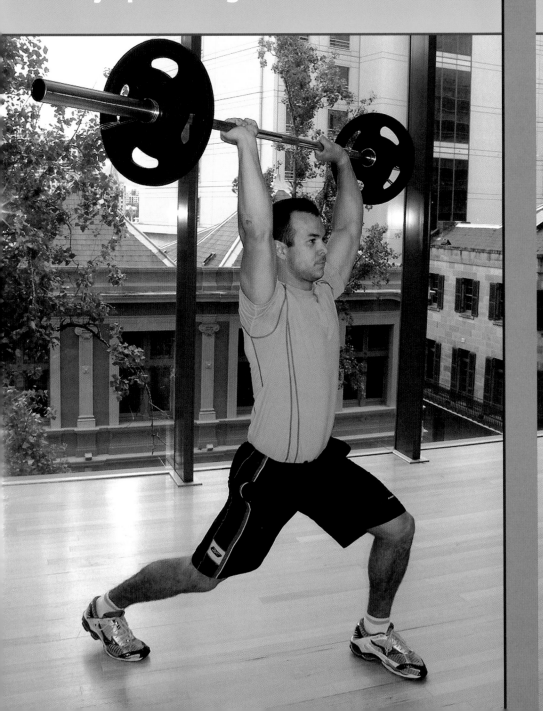

## Developing Explosive Power

To perform the lifts encountered in this chapter, you will have successfully progressed through training Phases 1-3. The progression element is critically important because along the way your body will have improved its core strength, mobility and neuromuscular capacity. You will have also exposed the connective tissues, tendons, ligaments and muscle fibers to various angles and degrees of resistance and speed which helps the body become more functional in sport, allowing it to cope with a variety of forces and activities, whilst also reducing one's risk of injury.

When learning an Olympic lift, it is essential that a major emphasis is placed on learning proper technique first using lighter weights. The goal is to increase power output which comes from moving a weight quickly. If the weight is too heavy, the bar will move slowly and the athlete's technique will suffer potentially causing injury. Over time as technique and speed improves, gradually the weight is increased on the bar, contributing to effective development of speed and power conversion.

As a coach, I understand the importance and benefits of Olympic lifting and the carryover to one's sport, through better coordination and developing a higher rate of force. Even if that ranges from the traditional Power Clean to the much more complex Snatch, Olympic lifts train the athlete to explode and use the maximum possible force. As a result, quality of movement is favored over quantity with longer rest breaks to ensure the body is fresh when performing lifts.

## Power Output

Upon reaching this point in strength training, we see a rapid increase in the power output incurred in each lift. The motor unit involvement will often depend upon the force output. The rapid development of force involving the mass and acceleration contributes to power and speed itself. I like to think Phase 4 involves two sub-power phases:

- **Power Phase 1:** light load (or weight) being lifted at high speed including medicine balls and Olympic lifts; ensuring mastery of technique; lift speed often used to imitate sport specific power performed at high velocity such as the Shot Put
- **Power Phase 2:** heavy load being lifted at high speed

Because of the rapid movements and muscle recruitment of these powerful lifts, the neural system is highly taxed requiring longer recovery periods between sets of 3-6 minutes. In between sets, light cardiovascular exercise (i.e. stationary bike) can be performed to assist in oxygen circulation and keeping muscles warm whilst also assisting later in the cooling down phase followed by stretching to reduce any muscle soreness.

Weights greater than 85-90% of your maximum will result in the greatest neural gains. Most athletes will only have the ability to handle these intensities for 1-3 repetitions and require more than 3-6 minutes recovery before repeating. Weights at around 75-85% of one's maximum can impact on both strength and neural gains with 4-8 reps and recovery of 3-5 minutes. Following a progressive strength training program provides the stimulus for your body to adapt to the power output and become more efficient as both the coordination and firing of muscles improves.

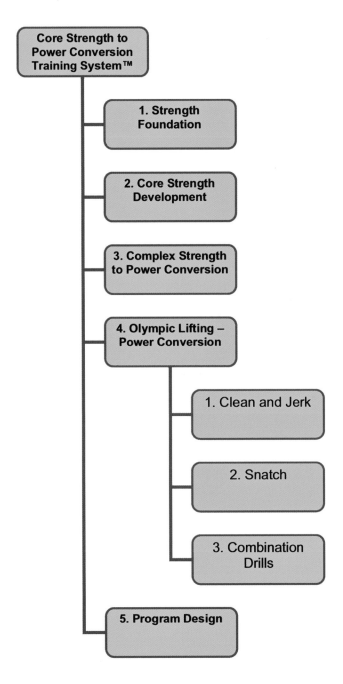

# Key Stretches for Olympic Lifts

Olympic lifting requires tremendous strength, mobility and stability of a joint to ensure correct movement technique is maintained at all times. On some occasions, special attention may need to be applied regularly to ensure this mobility is maintained. The following stretches target specific muscular groups utilized in Olympic lifts. Each stretch is held for up to 15 seconds or more and repeated on both sides of body, as required.

| Key Stretches | Description |
|---|---|

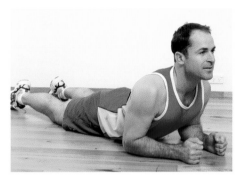

### Back Extension – elbows

**Objective:** Stretch lower back muscles, to assist with set-up and first pull phases.

Lie on ground on stomach and forearms and gently rise chest up off ground and hold without stress or pain.

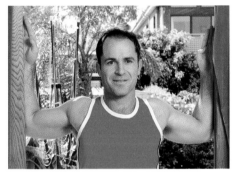

### Chest Stretch

**Objective:** Stretch chest muscles and assist in good body alignment, pulling movement and bar position, especially when overhead.

Stand between door frame (or corner of two walls – L-shape) with arms at 90-degrees and gently lean forwards.

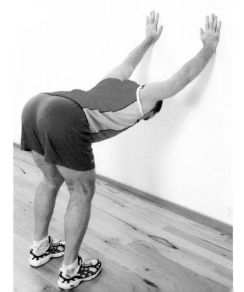

### Mid-Back Arch

**Objective:** Stretch mid and upper back and shoulder region to assist with the bar position, especially when overhead (i.e. Snatch).

Stand opposite to wall and between door frame (or corner of two walls – L-shape). Bend at hips, place hands on wall and gently lean forwards.

**Note:** Daily stretching and weekly massage is recommended.

### Triceps

**Objective:** Stretch upper back, scapula and triceps. Important in shoulder and scapula mobility in all upper body and overhead movements.

Bend arm behind head and grip elbow with opposite hand. Gently pull downwards. Repeat with opposite arm.

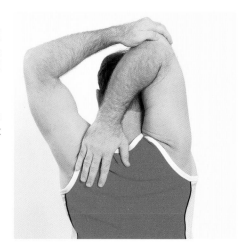

### Adductors

**Objective:** Stretch groin region to assist with rapid leg movement from bent to raised position and jerk movement pattern.

Sit on ground with soles of feet together and place forearms along legs, gripping ankles with hands. Gently push knees down towards grounds by using your arms, before relaxing.

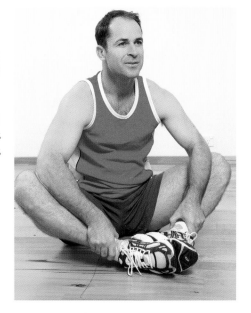

### Hamstrings

**Objective:** Stretch hamstrings muscles involved in squat movements.

Sit on ground with legs extended and one foot on top of the other. Extend arms behind the body with fingers cupped and pointed. Keeping spine long, gently lean forwards for stretch. Repeat with opposite leg.

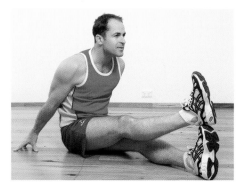

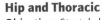

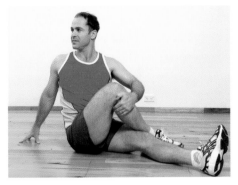

## Hip and Thoracic

**Objective:** Stretch hip and mid back region to ensure pliability of muscle for all movements.

Sit upright on floor with one leg extended and cross the other over and place foot on ground. Using the opposite arm, support the knee of the bent leg with your hand. Gently turn shoulders towards opposite knee for stretch with the other hand resting behind the body for support. Repeat stretch on opposite leg.

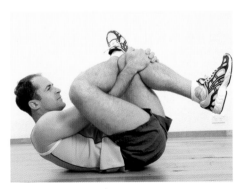

## Lumbar Rotation

**Objective:** Stretch hip, lower and mid back regions to ensure pliability of muscle for all movements.

Lie on ground with arms out wide and one leg bent across the other. Lower leg to side and face head across to other side. Repeat opposite direction.

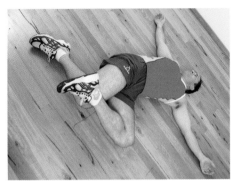

## Piriformis

**Objective:** Stretch deep gluteal muscles involved in all lower body movements.

From the above stretch, lean back onto ground and reach hand of bent leg through hole between legs and the other around outside of leg so both are placed just below knee and pull body close. Repeat opposite leg.

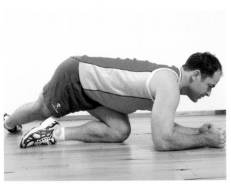

## Kneeling Sacroiliac Joint

**Objective:** Stretch deep gluteal muscles and sacroiliac joint involved in all lower body movements.

Kneel on ground and lean forwards onto forearms. Cross one leg behind the other keeping the hips square. Repeat opposite leg.

### Standing Thigh

**Objective:** Stretch thigh muscles involved in all squat, lunge and pull movements.

Standing tall, grab foot and bend up behind body and hold. Repeat opposite leg.

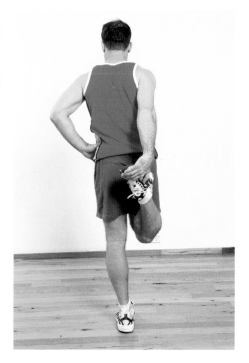

### Kneeling Side Reach

**Objective**: Stretch hip, thigh and back muscles used in all lifting movements. Kneel in lunge position with legs at 90-degrees. Gently lean forward and place forearm across forward leg. Raise rear arm into the air and gently bend legs and lean forward. Extend raised arm (and shoulder) slightly back and across for stretch. Repeat stretch on opposite side.

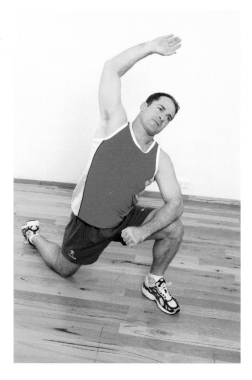

# 1. Clean and Jerk

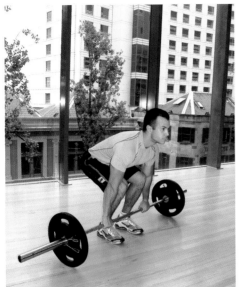

1. Start

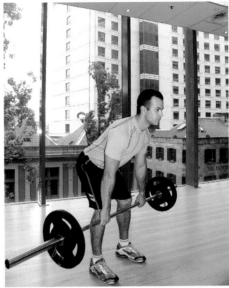

2. First Pull

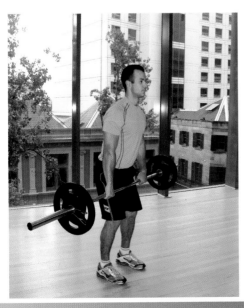

3. Scoop

4. Second Pull

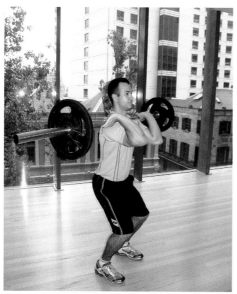

5. Descent under Bar

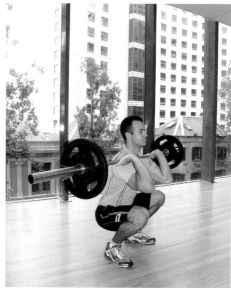

6. Catch

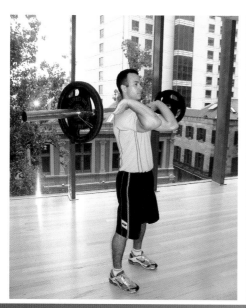

7. Finish

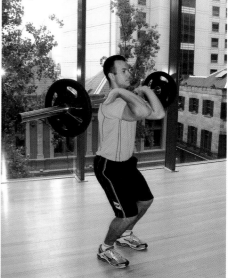

8. Knee and Hip Flexion

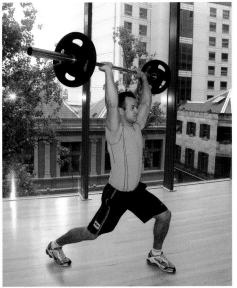

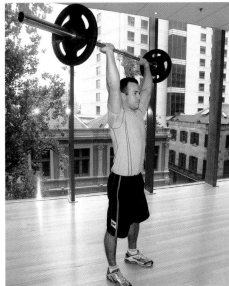

| 9. Extend and Catch | 10. Finish Position |

## Instruction

### 1. SET-UP

- Stand over barbell on Olympic platform or appropriate flooring with feet positioned under the bar slightly wider apart than hip width with toes slightly pointed outwards.
- Squat down and grip the bar with an overhand grip slightly wider than shoulder width.
- Position the shoulders over the bar and flatten back.
- Arms are straight with elbows pointed along the bar.

### 2. FIRST PULL

- Pull the bar up off the floor by extending the hips and knees.

### 3. SCOOP

- As the bar reaches the knees, vigorously raise the shoulders while keeping the barbell close to the thighs.
- When the barbell passes mid-thigh, allow it to contact the thighs.

### 4. SECOND PULL

- Drive upwards extending the body.
- Shrug the shoulders and pull the barbell upward with the arms allowing the elbows to flex out to the sides, keeping the bar close to the body.

### 5. DECENT UNDER BAR

- Aggressively pull the body under the bar, rotating the elbows around the bar.

## 6. CATCH
- Catch the bar on front of shoulders while lowering into a squat position.

## 7. FINISH
- Upon reaching full squat, stand up immediately.

## 8. KNEE AND HIP FLEXION
- Adjust grip if necessary.
- Inhale and position the chest high with torso region braced tightly.

## 9. EXTEND AND CATCH
- Keeping pressure on the heels, dip the body by bending the knees and ankles slightly.
- Explosively drive upward with the legs, driving the barbell up off the shoulders. Drop body downward and split one foot forward and the other backward as fast as possible while vigorously extending the arms overhead.
- The split position places the front shin vertical to the floor with the front foot flat on the floor. The rear knee is slightly bent with the rear foot positioned on the toes. The bar should be positioned directly over the ears at arm's length with the back straight.

## 10. FOOT RECOVERY AND FINISH POSITION
- Push up with both legs.
- Position feet side by side by bringing the front foot back partway and then the rear foot forward (depending on your coaching style).

Upon completion, drop the bar from the finish position overhead in front of body on the platform, whilst stepping back away before trapping, if necessary, to stop the bar's movement.

## 2. Snatch

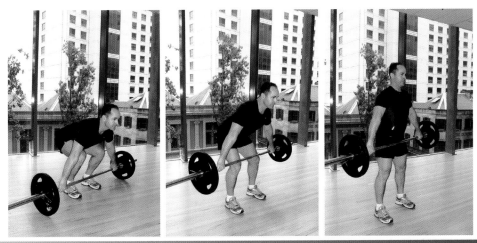

| 1. Start Position | 2. First Pull | 3. Scoop |

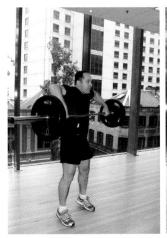 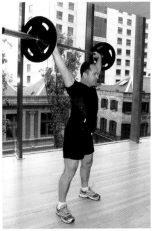

| 4. Second Pull | 5. Descent under Bar & Catch | 6. Finish Position |

### Instructions

#### 1. START POSITION
- Stand over barbell on Olympic platform or appropriate flooring with feet positioned under the bar slightly wider apart than hip width with toes slightly pointed outwards.
- Squat down and grip the bar with an overhand hook grip wider than shoulder width. (See Competition Snatch Phase 3 on page 124 for more details on wider arm position and Phase 1 on page 29 for hook grip description and illustrations.)
- Position the shoulders over the bar and arch back.
- Arms are straight with elbows pointed along the bar.

#### 2. FIRST PULL
- Pull the bar up off the floor by extending the hips and knees.

#### 3. SCOOP
- As the bar reaches the knees, the back stays arched and maintains a similar angle to the floor as in the starting position.
- As the barbell passes the knees, vigorously push the hips forward and raise the shoulders while keeping the bar as close to the legs as possible.
- As the bar passes the upper thighs, allow it to contact the thighs.

#### 4. SECOND PULL
- Drive upwards, extending the body by pushing off the calves.
- Shrug the shoulders and pull the barbell upward with the arms allowing the elbows to flex out to the sides, keeping the bar close to the body.
- Aggressively pull the body under the bar, rotating the elbows around the bar.

#### 5. DECENT UNDER BAR AND CATCH
- Catch the bar at arm's length while lowering into the squat position.

#### 6. FINISH POSITION
- As soon as the barbell is caught on the locked out arms in the squat position, squat up into standing position with barbell overhead.

Upon completion, drop the bar from the finish position overhead in front of body on the platform, whilst stepping back away before trapping, if necessary, to stop the bar's movement.

# 3. Combination Drills

In addition to specific Olympic lifts, in this section we combine multiple power drills for more advanced lifters looking for variety and additional training stimulus. Combination drills should only be attempted and performed after mastering exercises 1 and 2 in this chapter.

## a. Clean to Full Squat and Push Press

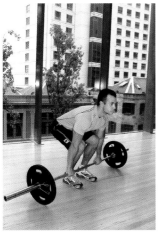

1. Start Position

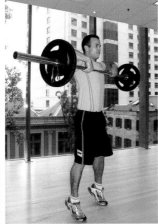

2. Pull & Scoop

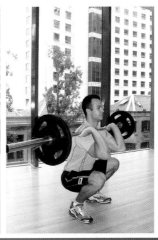

3. Descent under Bar & Catch

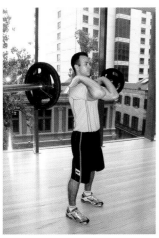

4. Rise

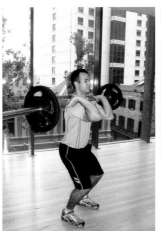

5. Dip

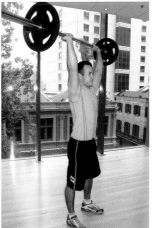

6. Finish Position

## b. Power Clean to Push Jerk

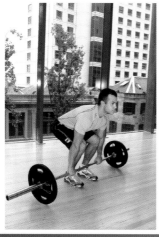
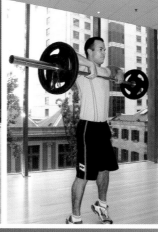
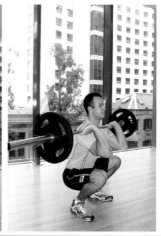

| 1. Start Position | 2. Pull & Scoop | 3. Descent under Bar & Catch |

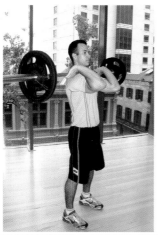
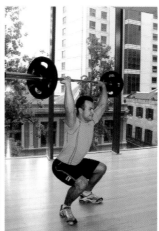
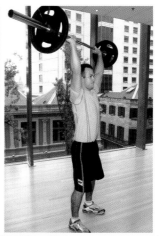

| 4. Rise | 5. Drop and Push | 6. Finish Position |

## c. Power Clean and Jerk

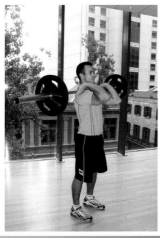
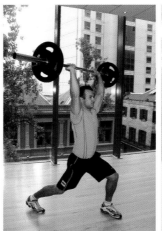
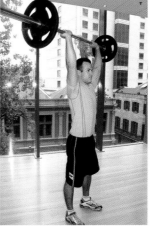

| 1. Start Position | 2. Pull & Scoop | 3. Descent under Bar & Catch |

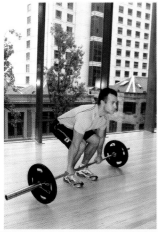
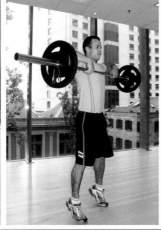
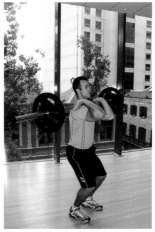

| 4. Rise | 5. Dip | 6. Finish Position |

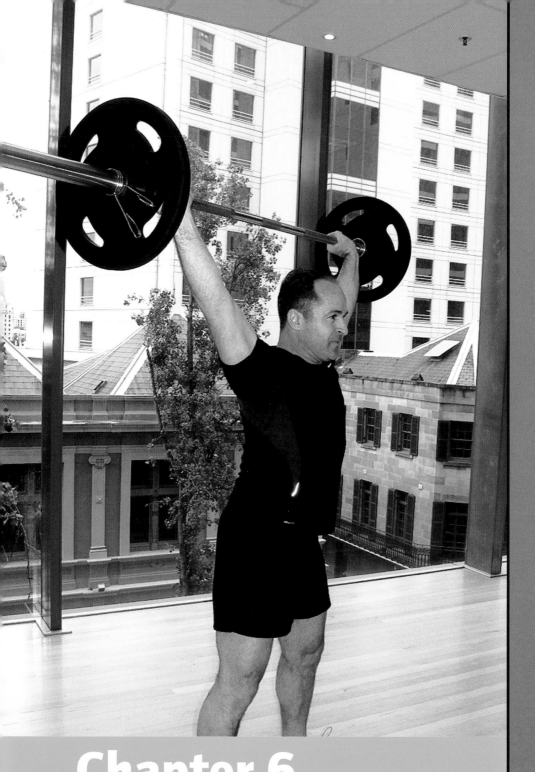

# Chapter 6
## Phase 5: Program Design

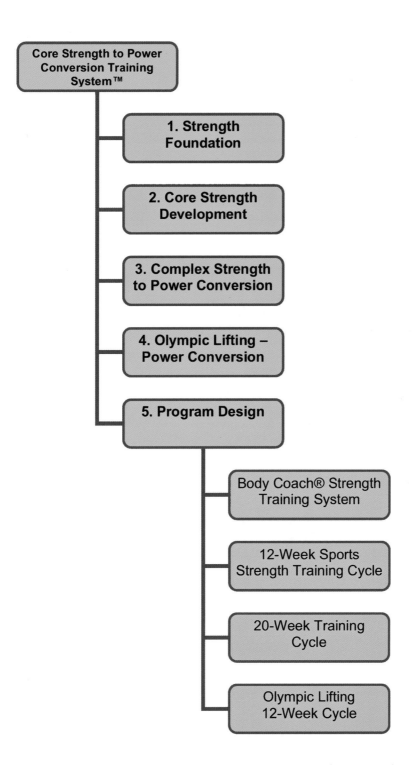

# Strength Training Routines

Strength training plays an important role in neuromuscular strength and coordination required for optimal athletic performance. In this chapter I will provide you with a number of strength training programs for sports and general fitness. The foundation for these programs is outlined in Chapter 2 page 19.

**To ensure safe progress with strength training, adhere to the following strength training guidelines:**

- Gain approval to exercise from your doctor, especially if you have a previous injury.

- See a Physical Therapist to assess your posture and joint mechanics and approve appropriate exercises for you.

- Have a Strength and Conditioning Coach demonstrate each exercise and correct any faults you may have whilst performing them yourself.

- Get to know your muscles to understand their function.

- Warm-up the body prior to exercising followed by pre-activity stretching.

- Ensure that the head and neck maintain neutral position in line with the lower back at all times.

- If at any stage during exercising you feel tension, numbness, dizziness or pain, stop the exercise immediately and seek medical advice.

- Warm up with 5-10 minutes of light cardiovascular exercise and stretches for the whole body.

- Emphasize quality of movement over quantity.

- Rest 60-180+ seconds between each set, as required.

- Drink at least 2 glasses of water during your workout, then afterwards.

- Give yourself at least 24-72 hours to recover before repeating for strength and power training respectively.

- Cool down with light cardiovascular exercise and gentle stretching routine after your workout.

- Apply strength training cycle to progress development (see graph).

**Note:** Refer to 8 Key Elements (page 19) as your training guide with each exercise.

# Starting Point

Sets and repetitions are the building blocks of your strength training routine. A repetition (or rep) is one complete execution of an exercise. So, for example, one rep of a squat exercise would be the full cycle squatting down and then back up. On the other hand, a set refers to a series of repetitions (i.e. 8 reps complete one set) followed by a recovery period. In scientific terms, a movement is often classified as eccentric (negative or down part) and concentric (positive or up part) such as that in a bench press or squat exercise. I mention these terms because over time you will hear a number of words in the gym or notice terms while reading used to describe an exercise or movement with similar meanings. In our case, my aim is to keep things as simple as possible.

Each repetition should also move through its full range of motion. In the case of the bench press exercise, this means pushing the weight up (concentric) until your arms are straight, then lowering it back down (eccentric) towards the chest without stopping. The specific number of sets and repetitions are determined by one's training objective as described in chapter 2.

A training cycle is generally applied over a 4-week period. For instance, the general preparation cycle may be performed over 4 weeks, before moving on to the strength cycle for 4 weeks and so forth. As strength and muscle coordination improves during this 4-week period, a small increase in the maximal percentage of weight being lifted can be applied or a new exercise for the same muscle group introduced.

In advanced training, percentiles are calculated by performing a one repetition maximum lift. But when first starting out, there is a period of 8-12 weeks where the body needs to adapt appropriately before these tests are undertaken – under the supervision of a qualified strength and conditioning coach. In the beginning, using a light weight that fulfills the required amount of reps will give you the starting point to build from as your knowledge and understanding increases. As the body adapts quickly and needs new variables, either the weight being lifted is increased, the tempo is changed, the recovery period is reduced or a new exercise for the same muscle group introduced – as per 8 Key Elements (page 19).

In strength training terms, progressive resistance training would mean lifting a heavier weight once your body has adjusted to the usual weight lifted. It is wise to first increase the number of repetitions and sets rather than increase the weight. Only once you have increased the repetitions and sets should you then look for further gains by increasing the weight. With repetition changes throughout the program – for example – from 10 to 12 reps or 8 to 10 reps, this may equate to a 5 or 10% increase in weight added to the exercise. A small increase in weight added may actually decrease the specified amount of reps allocated. This is when you gain a good understanding of your true training repetition range adapted into a strength cycle. Hence, when 12 repetitions of one exercise becomes easy for the 2-3 sets completed, a 5% increase may be added at your next training session. This 5% increase may result in a smaller amount of repetitions being performed in the final set, but that's okay because this is when the body really starts to work. The idea is to stay with this weight until this too becomes easy, then increase the weight again in small increments, whilst considering the speed ratio aspect. These ongoing changes never allow the body to adapt and changes in body shape and muscle tone will occur.

A basic beginner's routine consists of 1 to 3 sets for each major muscle group, with 10 to 15 reps performed per set. Between sets you rest for approximately 60–90 seconds or more, until you feel ready to tackle the exercise again. You'll require longer rests of 180 seconds or more between sets of more complex or higher intensity power exercises in the future. The rest period is also a great time to stretch or complete less strenuous exercises such as training the abdominal region to help maximize training time and drink some water to replenish the body.

Another rule of thumb in terms of rest relates to the amount of time before training the same muscle group again. It is recommended that once reps of less than 8-10 are being used at least 48 hours of rest time is required before training the same muscle groups again. Various research shows that training programs should limit periods of complete inactivity to no more than two to three weeks. Prolonged periods of inactivity should be avoided and the training program should incorporate some form of body maintenance training where a prolonged break is desired.

## Training Progression

Prior to starting any exercise in your program, always perform a very light warm-up set of the exercise to prepare you physically and mentally. Beginners should use slow, controlled movements with a continuous flow when starting out – avoid stopping – instead keep the movement flowing until all reps are completed. This keeps the muscle under tension for the whole set and is where real strength gains occur. Over many months of training the speed and power of the movement will increase due to the amount of weight being lifted. As a result, the neuromuscular function will also improve resulting in better muscle coordination and an increase in one's metabolic rate that leans up muscle tissue and burns fat more effectively.

When you are first starting out and figuring out what weights are good for you, you'll have to go through some trial and error to find the correct weight. It is my recommendation that before you start any exercise or training program that you seek your doctor's approval and train under the supervision of a qualified strength and conditioning coach to learn the exercises and train with good form. Essentially, lift a lighter weight for between 10 to 15 reps with good form. The 10 to 15 repetition range is based on the principle that beginners should use slightly lower weight for the first month, in order to allow their connective tissue, muscles and nervous system time to adapt to the loading.

## 1. Body Coach® Strength Training System

To assist in the development of strength training, for those who are looking for a simple training model to follow, I have developed the Body Coach® Strength Training System for the upper and lower body regions. The concept behind this system relates to having a program that targets all major muscle groups of the body yet allows you to pick and choose the exercises to perform from a selection supplied, or more if necessary. This provides you with plenty of variety as well as options when going to the gym and equipment isn't available or being used by another person – you can simply choose another exercise for the same muscle group without delay.

This system relates to Phases 1 and 2 – involving Strength Foundation and Core Strength Exercises. The exercises within each muscle group of the upper and lower body training systems are found within this book. Additional exercises may be included.

## Body Coach® Strength Training System Guidelines:

- Choose 2 exercises from each muscle group in upper body (or only 1 exercise in various lower body exercises) for example:
- CHEST: 1. Bench Press; 2: Incline Bench Press
- BACK:  1. Lat Pull down; 2. Single Arm Rows
- Perform 4 sets of 10-12 reps (12, 12, 10, 10) with 60 seconds rest between sets
- **4-week training cycle**: 3 days per week (i.e. Mon, Wed, Fri)

|          | Training Day 1 | Training Day 2 | Training Day 3 |
|----------|----------------|----------------|----------------|
| Week 1   | Upper Body     | Lower Body     | Upper Body     |
| Week 2   | Lower Body     | Upper Body     | Lower Body     |
| Week 3   | Upper Body     | Lower Body     | Upper Body     |
| Week 4   | Lower Body     | Upper Body     | Lower Body     |

- **4-week training cycle**: 2 days a week: Day 1: Upper Body; Day 2: Lower Body
- Refer to pages 19-69 for exercises.

## Body Coach® Upper Body Strength Training System

| | Exercise List | Reps | Sets | Rest | Weight |
|---|---|---|---|---|---|
| **Chest** | 1. Bench Press | 12 | 4 | 60 Seconds | |
| | 2. Incline Bench Press | 12 | | | |
| | 3. Dumbbell Bench Press – Flat | 10 | | | |
| | 4. Dumbbell Bench Press – Incline | 10 / 12 | 4 | 60 Seconds | |
| | 5. Dumbbell Flyes – Flat | 12 | | | |
| | 6. Dumbbell Flyes – Incline | 10 / 10 | | | |
| **Back** | 1. Lat Pulldown – Wide Grip | 12 | 4 | 60 Seconds | |
| | 2. Lat Pulldown – Reverse Grip | 12 | | | |
| | 3. High Bench Pulls | 10 / 10 | | | |
| | 4. Single Arm Rows | 12 / 12 | 4 | 60 Seconds | |
| | 5. Chin-ups – Wide Grip | 10 / 10 | | | |

| Muscle Group | Exercise | Reps | Sets | Rest |
|---|---|---|---|---|
| **Shoulders** | 1. Seated Front Shoulder Press | 12 | 4 | 60 Seconds |
| | 2. Seated Rear Shoulder Press | 12 10 10 | | |
| | 3. Standing Military Press | 12 12 | | |
| | 4. Lateral RaisesPush Press | 10 10 | | |
| **Biceps** | 1. Barbell Biceps Curl | 12 | 4 | 60 Seconds |
| | 2. Alternate Arm Biceps Curl | 12 10 10 | | |
| | 3. Seated Preacher Curl | 12 12 | | |
| | 4. Hammer Curl | 10 10 | | |
| **Triceps** | 1. Lying Triceps Extension | 12 | 4 | 60 Seconds |
| | 2. Arm Dips | 12 10 | | |
| | 3. Triceps Push Down | 10 | | |
| | 4. Standing Overhead Triceps Extension | 12 12 | | |
| | 5. Close Grip Bench Press | 10 10 | | |

**Note:**
- Choose 2 exercises for each muscle group.
- Add additional exercises for each muscle group, if necessary.
- Apply 4-week training cycle with 3:1:1 tempo.
- Apply second 4-week training cycle using 2 x 10 and 2 x 8 reps and modify tempo to: 2:1:1; rest for 90-seconds.
- See Chapter 2 for 8 Key Elements to consider.

## Body Coach® Lower Body Strength Training System

| Exercise List | Reps | Sets | Rest | Weight |
|---|---|---|---|---|
| **Choose 2 Exercises** | | | | |
| **Thigh/Butt** | | | | |
| 1. Leg Press | 12 | 4 | 60 Sconds | |
| 2. Single Leg Press | 12 | | | |
| 3. Front Squat | 10 | | | |
| 4. Squat | 10 | | | |
| 5. Stationary Lunges (Barbell) – Alternate Legs | 12 12 | | | |
| 6. Leg Extension | 10 | | | |
| 7. Single Leg Extension | 10 | | | |
| **Choose 1 Exercise** | | | | |
| **Hamstrings** | | | | |
| 1. Leg Curls | 12 12 | 4 | 60 Seconds | |
| 2. Single Leg Curls | 10 10 | | | |
| 3. Romanian Dead-Lift | 12 12 10 | | | |
| 4. Glute-Ham Holds | 10 | | | |
| **Choose 1 Exercise** | | | | |
| **Calves** | | | | |
| 1. Standing Calf Raise Off Step | 12 12 | 4 | 60 Seconds | |
| 2. Single Leg Standing Calf Raise Off Step Holding Dumbbell | 10 10 | | | |
| 3. Machine Standing Calf Raise | 12 12 10 | | | |
| 4. Seated Calf Raise | 10 | | | |

**10-15 Minute Workout:**

**Core/Abs**

1. Body Dish – Supine
2. Medicine Ball Raise
3. Fitness Ball Abdominal Crunch
4. Collins-Lateral Fly™ Series – Long Lever Holds
5. Collins-Lateral Fly™ Series – Coordination Drills

**Note:**
The abdominal and lower back muscles play a key role in posture and muscular synergy between the upper and lower body. As a result, spend up to 15 minutes performing exercises to strengthen this region using:
(a) Time on task (i.e. 30 seconds)

6. Lateral Side Raises
7. Medicine Ball Elbow to Knee
8. Lower Leg Lifts
9. Knee Raise
10. Hanging Knee Raises
11. Hip Raise – Shoulder Bridge
12. Controlled Back Raise

(b) Repetition Ratio – 3:1:1
(c) Refer to Phase 2; Core strength for sample program repetition guidance

**Note:**
- Add additional exercises for each muscle group, if necessary.
- Apply 4-week training cycle with 3:1:1 tempo.
- Apply second 4-week training cycle using 2 x 10 and 2 x 8 reps and modify tempo to: 2:1:1; rest for 90-seconds.
- See Chapter 2 for 8 Key Elements to consider.
- Refer to Phase 2: Core strength for repetition guidance.

# 2. 12-Week Sports Strength Training Cycle

Strength training is an essential part of any sports conditioning in order to reduce injury risk and optimize playing performance. The following 12-week Sports Strength Training Cycle is based upon athletes with a solid strength foundation already in place. Periods of strength development aim to improve maximum force production, whilst periods of power conversion aim to allow athletes to produce strength reserves in a much shorter time by becoming more powerful. The major benefit of the training approach that follows is the simple method that applies a Push, Pull and Squat approach requiring minimal equipment (barbell and flat bench) – which is great for smaller underfunded clubs world-wide and those with this equipment at home.

This training model is much more specific and based on contact sports that play over an extended period of time. For example: NFL, NHL, Rugby League, Rugby Union and similar. The following tables illustrate a 12-week training plan. On this occasion I will demonstrate overload and progression through the use of training loads at a relative percentage of one's 1RM. On each 4-week cycle the training load will decrease which allows adaptation to occur. This program is presented over 3 training days each week with intensity based as a percentage of maximum:

More technical Olympic lift progressions would be introduced when planning a second 12-week training cycle.

## Weeks 1 – 4

| Exercises Days 1 & 3 | Exercises Day 2 | Sets x Reps | | | | Rest (seconds) |
|---|---|---|---|---|---|---|
| | | W1 | W2 | W3 | W4 | |
| Squat | Romanian Dead-Lift | 4 x 12 | 4 x 10 | 4 x 10 | 3 x 12 | 90 |
| Bench Press | Straight Arm Shrug | 4 x 12 | 4 x 10 | 4 x 10 | 3 x 12 | 90 |
| Bent Over Row | Upright Row | 4 x 12 | 4 x 10 | 4 x 10 | 3 x 12 | 90 |
| Standing Military Press | Stationary Lunges | 4 x 12 | 4 x 10 | 4 x 10 | 3 x 12 | 90 |

| Week | Day 1: Monday | Day 2: Wednesday | Day 3: Friday |
|---|---|---|---|
| 1 | 65% | 65% | 65% |
| 2 | 70% | 70% | 65% |
| 3 | 75% | 75% | 70% |
| 4 | 70% | 70% | 65% |

## Note:
- Perform 2 sets on each leg for a total of 4 sets with Stationary Lunges.
- Each weight percentage would be rounded down to the nearest combined weight.

**Weeks 5 – 8**

| Exercises Days 1 & 3 | Exercises Day 2 | Sets x Reps | | | | Rest (seconds) |
|---|---|---|---|---|---|---|
| | | W5 | W6 | W7 | W8 | |
| Power Clean | High Pull | 4 x 5 | 4 x 5 | 4 x 5 | 4 x 5 | 120 |
| Squat | Romanian Dead-Lift | 4 x 5 | 4 x 5 | 4 x 5 | 4 x 5 | 120 |
| Bench Press | Push Press | 4 x 5 | 4 x 5 | 4 x 5 | 4 x 5 | 120 |
| Bent Over Row | Stationary Lunges | 4 x 5 | 4 x 5 | 4 x 5 | 4 x 5 | 120 |

| Week | Day 1: Monday | Day 2: Wednesday | Day 3: Friday |
|---|---|---|---|
| 1 | 80% | 80% | 85% |
| 2 | 82.5% | 82.5% | 77.5% |
| 3 | 85% | 85% | 80% |
| 4 | 82.5% | 82.5% | 77.5% |

Note:
- Perform 2 sets on each leg for a total of 4 sets with Stationary Lunges.
- Each weight percentage would be rounded down to the nearest combined weight.

**Weeks 9 – 12**

| Exercises Days 1 & 3 | Exercises Day 2 | Sets x Reps | | | | Rest (seconds) |
|---|---|---|---|---|---|---|
| | | W9 | W10 | W11 | W12 | |
| Power Clean | High Pull | 4 x 3 | 3 x 3 | 3 x 2 | 3 x 1 | 180+ |
| Squat | Romanian Dead-Lift | 4 x 3 | 3 x 3 | 3 x 2 | 3 x 1 | 180+ |
| Bench Press | Push Press | 4 x 3 | 3 x 3 | 3 x 2 | 3 x 1 | 180+ |
| Bent Over Row | Stationary Lunges | 4 x 3 | 3 x 3 | 3 x 2 | 3 x 1 | 180+ |

| Week | Day 1: Monday | Day 2: Wednesday | Day 3: Friday |
|---|---|---|---|
| 1 | 87.5% | 87.5% | 82.5% |
| 2 | 90% | 90% | 85% |
| 3 | 92.5% | 92.5% | 87.5% |
| 4 | Max Test | Max Test | Day off |

Note:
- Perform 2 sets on each leg for a total of 4 sets with Stationary Lunges.
- Each weight percentage would be rounded down to the nearest combined weight.

# 3. 20-Week Training Cycle

The following 20-week strength training cycle is progressive in nature and aimed at taking you through a journey – developing general strength before building muscle and then maximizing strength gains and transferring this into power. This 20-week cycle will help shape the way you train in the future by getting to know how your body and mind work together and respond to the training stimulus at hand. This is because this program provides you with a benchmark training framework for you to follow.

As you will discover through regular participation, this training cycle can be modified and adapted to suit your specific training needs – as the ultimate combination of reps, sets, tempo and exercises for each individual will vary as well as the force being generated through the mass being lifted and acceleration of each lift itself. Each stage of the 20-week program needs to be completed in the specified order to get the maximum benefit. So I implore you to go into this 20-week training cycle with a positive mind-set towards practical learning from which you can adapt any future training and modifications using a similar 'framework' to suit your specific needs.

## Training Overview

The program is based on two programs (Y & Z) for each training phase which are alternated each time you train. The number of times you perform these will depend upon your training schedule and availability each week. As a result, I have provided a 2, 3 and 4-day training model below.

Each program is set out with the respective weeks at the top of the program. For example; if you can only train 2 days a week then this may entail Monday and Thursdays; 3 days a week – Monday, Wednesday and Friday; or 4 days a week – Monday, Tuesday, Thursday, Friday or similar. The training cycle requires you to complete all the specified sets of one exercise before moving on to the next exercise as this will help you achieve the goals of the program.

To achieve the most from your training, it is recommended that on your last set of any given exercise, you lift the heaviest weight possible for that number of repetitions. If you can complete all the repetitions specified in your last set, then you may need to increase the weights by 2.5 to 5%. As you progress through each cycle, a decrease in repetitions generally means an increase in weight. For instance, the weight you can lift for eight repetitions should be considerably heavier than what you can lift for ten. On some occasions though, the weight may be similar depending on the lifting tempo or the speed (see page 19) at which you perform the various phases of an exercise, so adapt accordingly. Here's one example of this using a bench press exercise when changing stages:

**Stage:** Hypertrophy
**Exercise:** Bench Press
**Lifting Tempo:** 3:1:3 – Lower the bar over a count of three seconds, pause for one second and then lift the weight up again over three seconds.

**Stage:** Strength
**Exercise:** Bench Press
**Lifting Tempo:** 2:1:1 – Lower the bar over a count of two seconds, pause for one second and then explode the weight up as fast as possible.

The time you take between sets is dependent on the program you are undertaking. Throughout each stage, the following rest between sets is recommended:
General Preparation: 60-90 seconds
Hypertrophy: 90 seconds
Max. Strength and Power: More than 180 seconds (3 minutes+)

## Training Tables

### 2 Training Sessions per Week

| Week | 1 | | 2 | | 3 | | 4 | |
|------|---|---|---|---|---|---|---|---|
| Session | 1 | 2 | 1 | 2 | 1 | 2 | 1 | 2 |
| Program | Y | Z | Y | Z | Y | Z | Y | Z |

### 3 Training Sessions per Week

| Week | 1 | | | 2 | | | 3 | | | 4 | | |
|------|---|---|---|---|---|---|---|---|---|---|---|---|
| Session | 1 | 2 | 3 | 1 | 2 | 3 | 1 | 2 | 3 | 1 | 2 | 3 |
| Program | Y | Z | Y | Z | Y | Z | Y | Z | Y | Z | Y | Z |

### 4 Training Sessions per Week

| Week | 1 | | | | 2 | | | | 3 | | | | 4 | | | |
|------|---|---|---|---|---|---|---|---|---|---|---|---|---|---|---|---|
| Session | 1 | 2 | 3 | 4 | 1 | 2 | 3 | 4 | 1 | 2 | 3 | 4 | 1 | 2 | 3 | 4 |
| Program | Y | Z | Y | Z | Y | Z | Y | Z | Y | Z | Y | Z | Y | Z | Y | Z |

# Training Program

Refer to training tables for application to 2, 3 or 4 sessions a week in the following stages in terms of performing Programs Y or Z.

### Stage 1 (weeks 1–4): General Preparation

| Program Y | Program Z | Sets x x Reps | Tempo | Rest (secs) |
|---|---|---|---|---|
| Leg Press | Bench Press | 3 x 15 | 2:1:2 | 60-90 |
| Lat Pull Down – Front | Incline Bench Press | 3 x 15 | 2:1:2 | 60-90 |
| Half-Squat | Single Arm Rows | 3 x 15 | 2:1:2 | 60-90 |
| Seated Row | Seated Shoulder Press | 3 x 15 | 2:1:2 | 60-90 |
| Leg Extension | Upright Rows | 3 x 15 | 2:1:2 | 60-90 |
| Barbell Biceps Curl | Lateral Raises | 3 x 15 | 2:1:2 | 60-90 |
| Hamstrings Curl | Triceps Push Down | 3 x 15 | 2:1:2 | 60-90 |

### Stage 2 (weeks 5–8): Hypertrophy

| Program Y | Program Z | Sets x x Reps | Tempo | Rest (secs) |
|---|---|---|---|---|
| Dead Lifts | Bench Press | 3 x 12 | 3:1:3 | 90 |
| Front Squats | Dumbbell Chest Flyes | 3 x 12 | 3:1:3 | 90 |
| Stationary Lunges | Seated Shoulder Press | 3 x 12 | 3:1:3 | 90 |
| Lat Pull Down | Lateral Raises | 3 x 12 | 3:1:3 | 90 |
| Bent Over Row | Lying Triceps Extension | 3 x 12 | 3:1:3 | 90 |
| Biceps Curl | Arm Dips | 3 x 12 | 3:1:3 | 90 |
| Alternate Arm Curl | Back Raises | 3 x 12 | 3:1:3 | 90 |

### Stage 3 (weeks 9–12): Strength

| Program Y | Program Z | Sets x x Reps | Tempo | Rest (secs) |
|---|---|---|---|---|
| Romanian Dead-Lifts | Bench Press | 4 x 10 | 2:1:2 | 90-120 |
| Front Squats | Incline Bench Press | 4 x 10 | 2:1:2 | 90-120 |
| Single Leg Press | Seated Shoulder Press | 4 x 10 | 2:1:2 | 90-120 |
| Lat Pull Down | Lateral Raises | 4 x 10 | 2:1:2 | 90-120 |
| Bent Over Row | Upright Row | 4 x 10 | 2:1:2 | 90-120 |
| Barbell Biceps Curl | Overhead Triceps Ext. | 4 x 10 | 2:1:2 | 90-120 |

### Stage 4 (weeks 13–16): Strength Conversion

| Program Y | Program Z | Sets x x Reps | Tempo | Rest (secs) |
|---|---|---|---|---|
| High Pulls | Split Jerk | 4 x 6 | Explosive | 180+ |
| Push Press | Bench Press | 4 x 6 | 2:1:1 | 180+ |
| Bent Over Rows | Incline Flyes | 4 x 6 | 2:1:1 | 180+ |
| Step Ups | Military Press | 4 x 6 | 2:1:1 | 180+ |
| Squats | Lateral Raises | 4 x 6 | 2:1:1 | 180+ |
| Dumbbell Rows | Lying Triceps Extension | 4 x 6 | 2:1:1 | 180+ |

### Stage 5 (weeks 17–20): Power Conversion

| Program Y | Program Z | Sets x x Reps | Tempo | Rest (secs) |
|---|---|---|---|---|
| High Pulls | Power Cleans | 4 x 3 | Explosive | 180+ |
| Push Press | Hang Snatch | 4 x 3 | Explosive | 180+ |
| Dead-Lift | Squat | 4 x 3 | 2:1:1 | 180+ |
| High Bench Pulls | Bench Press | 4 x 3 | 2:1:1 | 180+ |

Note: Abdominal exercises are performed in addition to this training program. See Phase 2 on core strength for specific exercises and sample training routine on page 87.

# 4. Olympic Lifting – 12-Week Cycle

## Cycle 1: Basic Lifts

All newcomers to Olympic lifts should progress through Phases 1-5 sequentially in order to fully understand the training progressions and lifts. The following 3 cycles themselves provide a basic lifts outline that focuses on 4 sets of 5 reps per exercise with exercises from this book specifically on improving Olympic lifts. The progression through each set is based on a pyramid approach that gradually increases the weight being lifted each set – light, medium, heavy over the 4 sets. As you progress in skill and understanding, a percentage of 1RM can be used and applied as seen in the 12-week sports strength cycle as well as managing the total volume of lifts being performed. Additional abdominal and medicine ball exercises are used to strengthen the core and increase neural adaptations for each stage are found in Phase 2 on page 71. Stage 1 should be performed a minimum of 2 or more days a week, with a day's rest in between.

### Cycle 1 (weeks 1–4): Basic Lifts

| Program A | Program B | Sets x x Reps | Tempo | Rest (secs) |
|---|---|---|---|---|
| Front Squat | Back Squat | 4 x 5 | 180+ | |
| Dead-Lift | Snatch Grip Dead-Lift | 4 x 5 | 180+ | |
| Standing Rear Shoulder Press | Press Behind Neck – Snatch Grip | 4 x 5 | 180+ | |

## Cycle 2: Lift Conversion

As you progress from 2-3 training sessions per week over a 4-week period with gradually increasing resistance, the aim is to gradually implement lift conversion exercises that are a modification of the complete Olympic lift as found in Phase 3.

### Cycle 2 (weeks 5-8): Lift Conversion

| Program A | Program B | Program C | Sets x Reps | Rest (secs) |
|---|---|---|---|---|
| Hang Clean | Hang Snatch | Hang Clean | 4 x 5 | 180+ |
| Press Behind Neck | Press Behind Neck – Snatch Grip | Push Press – Behind Neck | 4 x 5 | 180+ |
| Front Squat | Back Squat | Front Squat | 4 x 5 | 180+ |
| | | Dead-Lift | 4 x 5 | 180+ |

## Cycle 3: Power Conversion

The final 4-week cycle focuses on progressions of exercises from cycle 2 into full lifting patterns. This succession increases the power output of the exercises and requires total focus ensuring technique is maintained at all times. At the same time, specific strength exercises are maintained for continual development of support structures required in lifting.

### Cycle 2 (weeks 5-8): Power Conversion

| Program A | Program B | Program C | Sets x Reps | Rest (secs) |
|-----------|-----------|-----------|-------------|-------------|
| Power Clean | Power Snatch | Power Clean | 4 x 5 | 180+ |
| Power Jerk | Power Jerk | Overhead Squat | 4 x 5 | 180+ |
| Front Squat | Back Squat | Front Squat | 4 x 5 | 180+ |
| | | Dead-Lift | 4 x 5 | 180+ |

## Overview

Ultimately, there are multiple training cycles and strength and power training methods that can be applied. My goal as a coach has been to provide you with a practical strength foundation to build upon in the future. Athletes and coaches who participate in this program will gain both the theoretical and practical knowledge and understanding for optimal strength and power gains, then adapt this to best suit one's training needs. Think of it like learning how to drive with the assistance of a driving instructor. The more you practice and learn along the way, the better you'll become. Once you gain that valuable experience and start to improve your technique and spatial awareness, with confidence you will pass the driving test. In transferring this vision to *Strength Training for Men* you will have gained the vital practical experience and intramuscular coordination to adapt a specific training plan to suit you in the future. My personal goal was helping you reach this point.

My personal goal was helping you reach this point. In saying this, general hypertrophy training is important to increase the force-generation capacities of all muscles, as well as strengthening core muscles. This progresses into developing one's neural activation capacity of the relevant muscular framework in performing Olympic lifts. For those of you focused on sports improvements, just remember the maximization of transfer to sports performance requires the conversion of powerful muscles to a specific co-coordinated sports skill, thus the importance of including powerful Plyometric type drills found in my book titled: Power Training.

Time in training week-in and week-out must now also be devoted to injury prevention and body management including stretching, massage, physical therapy, chiropractic or similar as well as sound nutritional practices for optimal results.

I have enjoyed working with you and look forward to you achieving great results!

Paul Collins, The Body Coach®
**Australia's Personal Trainer™**
**www.thebodycoach.com**

# Appendix:
## Nutrient Timing for Optimal Strength, Muscle Growth and Power Gains

A number of athletes falter in their training, not in the gym itself, but the mechanism that replenishes the muscle and energy systems of the body during and immediately after this training period. Strength and power training combined with proper nutritional and supplemental balance is vital in maximizing ones performance gains.

During growth and strength phases, you may require supplements that support energy production such as Creatine and Glutamine as well as Glucosamine for protecting the joints, especially when you're lifting heavy. In addition, with the muscular disruption from strength and power training, to help reduce muscular breakdown and provide greater build-up, supplements such as Branched-Chain Amino Acids (BCAA's) and HMB have become the benchmark, in addition to ensuring optimal nutritional gains are supplied by whole foods and liquids including – water as well as carbohydrate and protein mixes and low fat milk.

The branched-chain amino acids (BCAAs) are Leucine, Isoleucine and Valine. In many fitness and sporting arenas, BCAAs seem to have been pushed aside in favor of Creatine and other similar products for muscle growth. Whilst Creatine is a great product, it has no effect on human protein synthesis rates after resistance exercise, whereas the anabolic effect of BCAAs on muscle growth, protein synthesis and recovery is unquestionable.

BCAAs are needed for the maintenance of muscle tissue and appear to preserve muscle stores of glycogen (a storage form of carbohydrate that can be converted into energy). BCAAs also help prevent muscle protein breakdown during exercise. BCAAs have an advantage for someone who wants to add muscle and who's dieting, as they have minimal calories, they're metabolized strictly in muscle and they're highly anabolic. Of all three BCAAs, leucine appears to be the most important for stimulating protein.

The table on the follwing page is an example only of what an elite athlete may use as a plan for enhancing optimal gains before, during and after training. Always see a sports nutritionist for supplements suitable for you.

| Moment | Phase | Time | Type* – Athletes over 18 years |
|---|---|---|---|
| Pre-Activity 1 | Energy | 1-3 hours before training | Whole food ingestion – depending on time of day (i. e. breakfast, lunch or dinner). Ensure a balance of carbs and protein with each meal. |
| Pre-Activity 2 | Energy | Example: on the way to gym | Amino acid/carbohydrate beverage such as Leucine enriched carbohydrate drink. (Creatine and HMB is often included depending on training cycle) |
| During Activity | Anabolic | Whilst training | 3:1-4:1 Carb:Protein ratio – Carbohydrate beverage enhanced with BCAA |
| Immediate Post Activity | Growth 1 | 0-45 minutes after training | 3:1-4:1 Carb:Protein ratio – Carbohydrate beverage enhanced with BCAA (Creatine and HMB is often included depending on training cycle.) |
| Late Post Activity | Growth 2 | Between 45 minutes and to 2 hours after training | Whole food ingestion – carbohydrate, protein and fat |
| In-between Training Bouts | Maintenance | Part of daily meal plan | 1. Daily meal plan - whole food ingestion 2. Protein shakes 3. Water 4. Vitamin supplements |

One of the most important things to remember is that sports supplements are secondary to nutritional whole foods. Their objective is aimed at supporting whole foods and assisting ones ability to train harder, recover quicker and perform at your optimal level all year round.
Various carb/Protein ratios will vary depending on specific training goals. If in doubt, try lactose free, low-fat milk as an affordable alternative to the above table.

*In terms of ones overall training, always consult a sports nutritionist for optimal nutritional planning supporting ones calorie intake, energy needs and supplement requirements including knowledge and understanding of specific types, amounts and timing. Be aware of a trial and error period to see how various food, liquids and supplements are handled by your body as every person is unique in the way they respond to them.

# Strength Training Index

# Phase 2:
# Core Strength Development 70

# Phase 3: Complex Strength to Power Conversion 88

# Body Coach® Education, Training & Products

Join The Body Coach® Paul Collins, international author and Strength and Conditioning Coach and his team of experts in the Fastfeet® Speed for Sport Training clinics, workshops, camps, seminars and coaching for all sports.

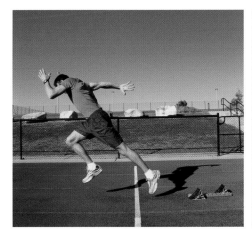 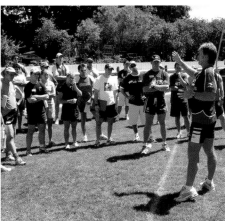

Paul Collins and Ron Palmer presenting Speed for Sport Coaching Seminar in Australia

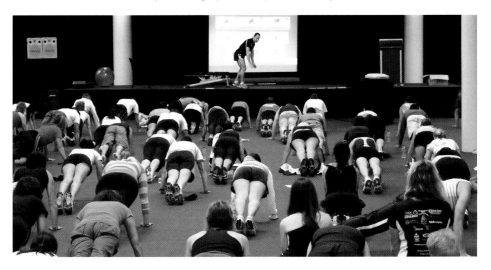

Paul presenting at International Fitness Conference, Sydney, Australia
For more details and products visit the following websites:

www.thebodycoach.com
www.bodycoach.com.au
www.fastfeet.com.au

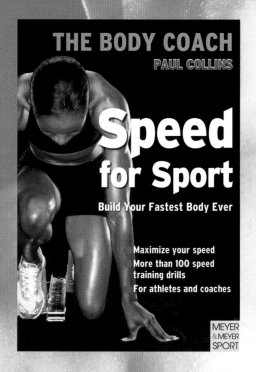
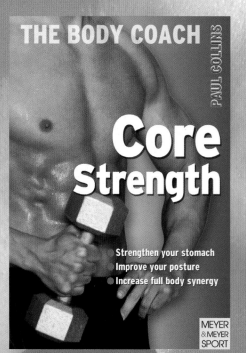

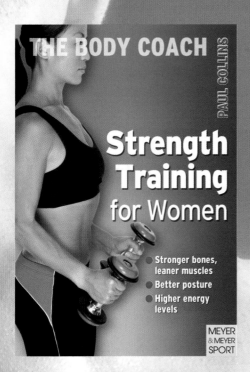

Paul Collins
**Strength Training for Women**

The combination of strength training, aerobic exercise and healthy eating habits has proven to be most effective for fat loss and muscle toning. *Strength Training* for Women has been developed as a training guide as more women begin to understand the health benefits of this activity. A series of strength training routines for use in the gym as well as a body weight workout routine that can be performed at home are included.

144 pages, full-color print
200 color photos
Paperback, $6^1/2''$ x $9^1/4''$
ISBN: 978-1-84126-248-2
$ 14.95 US / $ 22.95 AUS
£ 9.95 UK/€ 14.95

Paul Collins
**Functional Fitness**

*Functional Fitness* features practical, easy-to-follow exercises for athletes, coaches and fitness enthusiasts in helping build your fittest body ever by simulating sports-specific and daily lifestyle movement patterns. The Body Coach®, Paul Collins, provides step-by-step coaching and workouts utilizing: body weight, fitness balls, medicine balls, plyometrics, resistance bands, stability training and speed training equipment.

144 pages, full-color print
332 photos, 9 illustr., 3 charts
Paperback, $6^1/2''$ x $9^1/4''$
ISBN: 978-1-84126-260-4
$ 17.95 US / $ 29.95 AUS
£ 12.95 UK/€ 16.95

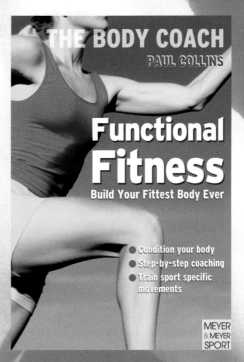

photos: Blende64 © Fotolia.com

MEYER & MEYER Sport | www.m-m-sports.com
sales@m-m-sports.com

MEYER
& MEYER
SPORT

Paul Collins
**Awesome Abs**

The abdominal muscles serve a critical function in daily movement, sport and physical activity. A strong mid-section helps support and protect your lower back region from injury. Is packed with over 70 easy-to-follow exercises and tests aimed at achieving a leaner abdomen, a stronger lower back, better posture and a trimmer waistline. You'll not only look and feel better, but athletes will find that a well-conditioned mid-section allows them to change direction faster, generate force quicker and absorb blows better.

136 pages, full-color print
229 photos & 4 illustrations
Paperback, $6^1/2$" x $9^1/4$"
ISBN: 978-1-84126-232-1
$ 14.95 US / $ 22.95 AUS
£ 9.95 UK/€ 14.95

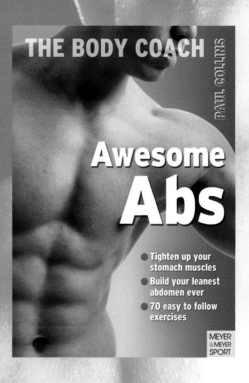

Paul Collins
**Power Training**

For many years, coaches and athletes have sought to improve power, a combination of speed and strength, in order to enhance performance. *Power Training* is designed as an educational tool to assist in the development of training programs that aim to keep athletes fit, strong and powerful all year round. 80 power training drills, tests and training routines are included which have also been used by Olympic and world class athletes to improve their performance. *Power Training* is an excellent guide for conditioned athletes to increase and develop their jumping, sprinting and explosive power.

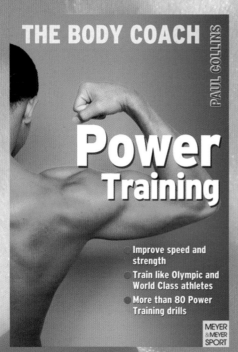

136 pages, full-color print
247 photos
Paperback, $6^1/2$" x $9^1/4$"
ISBN: 978-1-84126-233-8
$ 14.95 US / $ 22.95 AUS
£ 9.95 UK/€ 14.95

MEYER & MEYER Sport | www.m-m-sports.com
sales@m-m-sports.com

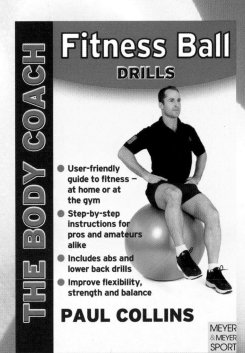

**Photo & Illustration Credits:**
Cover Photos: © fotolia ∕ © fotolia, pixel
Cover Design: Sabine Groten
Photos: Paul Collins